V.Q.E

THE TALE OF AN INDIAN PHYSICIAN IN THE UNITED KINGDOM OF 1980'S

VIVEK V GUMASTE

notionpress.com

Notion Press

Old No. 38, New No. 6
McNichols Road, Chetpet
Chennai - 600 031

First Published by Notion Press 2018

ISBN 978-1-64467-978-4

The traveler has to knock at every alien door to come to his own, and one has to wander through all the outer worlds to reach the innermost shrine at the end.

—Rabindranath Tagore, *Gitanjali*

Dedicated to those Indian Physicians who left their country for good or bad to further their careers and the travails that they faced in their efforts to attain professional satisfaction.

ABOUT THE TITLE: V.Q.E is an abbreviation for Visa Qualifying Exam: the rigorous and challenging test that foreign medical graduates had to pass to gain entry to practice medicine in the United States in the 1980's.

Contents

Contents

Preface

In 1980, after completing medical school in India, I landed in Britain to appear for the Visa Qualifying Exam (V.Q.E) in pursuit of my dream to get to the United States. I was young, a full 26 years old, ambitious and opinionated. The two and a half years that I spent in Britain were eventful.

My book is a recollection of those memories of Britain and my experience of that country. It is also a narrative of an ex-colonial subject coming face to face with the country of his ex-rulers and the bitterness that he feels toward Britain, the country that exploited his people. Additionally, it is a commentary on the travails faced by young foreign doctors as they go about advancing their careers in Britain. Thrown into this unlikely cocktail is the political backdrop of Britain in the 80s, the rise of Margaret Thatcher, the royal wedding of Princess Diana and Prince Charles, the Falklands War and British racism.

To what genre does this book belong? I am not sure. Is it a pristine memoir? Not exactly. Is it outright fiction? Certainly not. I would feel more comfortable in calling this book a quasi-factual reminiscence. Parts of my narration may not be one hundred percent accurate as I have depended on my memory to recall events that occurred more than 30 years ago. And I have used artistic license to embellish the written description of some of the personalities that figure in my account. However, the central theme of this story is authentic, the cardinal events recalled are true, and the feelings expressed are honest.

Prologue

I would be dishonest if I said that I disliked Great Britain. I didn't. "Dislike" was an understatement. I abhorred it with the full gravitas of the word; visceral disgust is another term that could approximate my true feelings. Having been born in India in 1954, a mere seven years after the British reluctantly parted with the country, and growing up at a time when the memory of a dominated nation was still fresh in the minds of Indians, I, naturally, harbored an animosity towards Britain as a nation and the English as a people.

Nevertheless, here I was, about to set foot in that very country. My passage to Britain was not a journey of choice, as it was for many awestruck sycophantic Indians of my era. Yes, at that time India had many Indians who, unlike me, looked up to Britain. It was a place that they admired; a fantasyland that made dreams come true for poor Third World Indians; a land of milk and honey that would make them rich beyond their wildest Indian aspirations. Mesmerized by this glowing idyll of Great Britain, they failed to appreciate the dark underbelly of the British and the atrocities they had committed in India – or rather, they chose to knowingly ignore it. What they saw instead was the "the proper Englishman," a superior human being who came from a more advanced land, his smart Western clothes, his well-articulated language and his white skin, all of which had been carefully projected to highlight the Indian's own inadequacy.

For the longest time, the word foreign (or *phoren*as the Indians pronounced it) was synonymous with Britain for most Indians. Their concept of an alien land began and ended with England, the commonly used term for Britain. Most Indians had little knowledge of other Western countries. The "States" did pop up occasionally in their soirees but was never a strong contender to usurp England's pride of place. In my case, opportunistic though it may sound but honest nevertheless, this trip was to be a stepping stone in my medical career with the lodestar being a little further away across the Atlantic, the United States of America, a country that represented the pinnacle of progress in the twentieth century.

The US to me was a country which reflected the best of mankind in modern times, a country that was wedded to liberty and equality, a country that was courageous enough to accept and confront the demons of its past, such as slavery, which Britain had never done. Abraham Lincoln's soul-stirring invocation, "Four score and seven years ago our fathers brought forth on this continent, a new nation, conceived in Liberty, and dedicated to the proposition that all men are created equal" had been my favorite speech in high school elocution contests.

The US was a nation that had risen to greatness not on the backs of colonial subjects, not by exploiting the resources of weaker nations but on its own merit and own diligence. That was where I was headed to further my medical career.

Unfortunately there was a stumbling block in my path. The Indian medical degree, MBBS, an acronym for Bachelor of Medicine and Bachelor of Surgery, (the jumbled sequence of the letters is due to its Latin origin, Medicinae Baccalaureus et Baccalaureus Chirurgiae) was not recognized in either the UK or the US. Therefore, in order to practice medicine in these countries, a fully trained physician from India had to be vetted by local boards through qualifying exams.

In the case of the US, the requisite exam went by the abbreviation ECFMG; ECFMG standing for Educational Commission for Foreign Medical Graduates, the designated certifying agency located in Philadelphia which was entrusted with the task of conducting certifying exams that regulated the flow of foreign physicians into the US.

The format of testing has undergone several transformations over the years. The process is rigorous and extensive. Initially it was a one-day six-hour long qualifying exam called the ECFMG exam. Later, in the 80s, the process was changed to a more extensive interrogation of one's medical knowledge, called the Visa Qualifying Exam (VQE) and was extended to two nerve-wracking days. In its latest avatar, it goes by the name of United States Medical Licensing Examination (USMLE) and consists of three parts that include a practical clinical component.

The list of testing locales has waxed and waned over the years. In the 60s and 70s ECFMG had several exam centers in India. Fearing a brain drain in the form of an exodus of medical professionals from the country, the Indian government did away with these native centers forcing thousands of Indian medical graduates to travel to Manila, Karachi or London (the closest centers to India) to take this exam.

Foreign travel for an Indian at that time was a prohibitive affair and beyond the reach of most middle-class families. A one-way ticket from Bombay (now Mumbai) to London or Manila could easily sap the entire life savings of a middle-class family. A trip for the express purpose of taking the exam was therefore out of question, being too risky and expensive.

It was then that I thought - why not travel to the UK and work there temporarily? This would fulfill my pecuniary needs and overcome the logistic hurdle of getting to an ECFMG exam center. Entry into the UK medical system was relatively easier. It did not involve complex visa issues. One could obtain a job almost immediately after passing the local certifying exam called Professional and Linguistic Assessment Board (PLAB).

That decision was however fraught with questions of social acceptability, and the very thought gave me butterflies in my stomach. British colonialism had infused in us Indians an inferiority complex. We were made to feel inferior in every way. Physically we were not as strong as the British; we were cowards when compared to the 'courageous' Englishman. Our culture was primitive, our history was irrelevant, our languages including Sanskrit, considered by many scholars to be the mother of all Indo-European languages, was no match for English, and our education was as good as nonexistent – this was the line that had been fed to us for nearly two hundred years.

Lord Thomas Macaulay (1800–1859) a British reformer in an address to the British parliament once remarked:

> "*It is, I believe, no exaggeration to say, that all the historical information which has been collected from all the books written in the Sanscrit language is less valuable than what may be found in the most paltry abridgements used at preparatory schools in England.*
>
> *All parties seem to be agreed on one point, that the dialects commonly spoken among the natives of this part of India, contain neither literary nor*

> *scientific information, and are, moreover, so poor and rude that, until they are enriched from some other quarter, it will not be easy to translate any valuable work into them.*"

The mantra that the British kept drumming into our heads was that the Raj was altruistic, not exploitative. The British being a superior people were duty-bound to reform the backward natives, was the idea that was propagated for universal consumption; a notion explicitly expressed in Rudyard Kipling's poem, *The White Man's Burden*:

> Take up the White Man's burden
> Send forth the best ye breed
> Go,bind your sons to exile
> To serve your captives' need;
> On fluttered folk and wild-
> Your new-caught sullen peoples,
> Half-devil and half child

Against this background, it was natural for me to experience a sense of social trepidation despite robust feelings about my own identity as an Indian. I wondered how I would fit into this new environment. Would I be able to adjust to the new lifestyle? How would I interact with the British people?

And on that note of apprehension, and unease, my journey to appear for the VQE began.

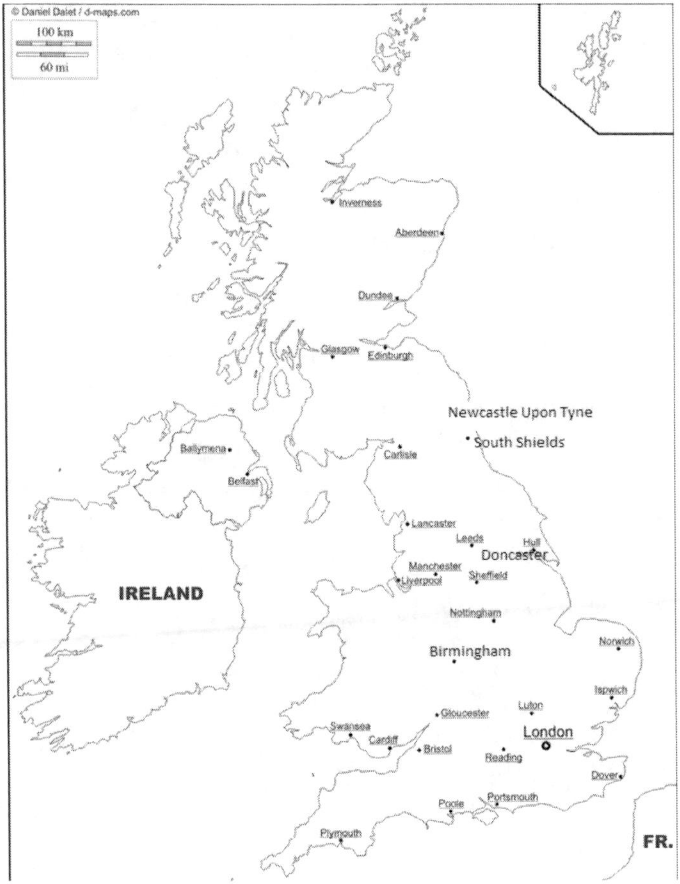

Fig.1:Map of the United Kingdom

The Physician Hierarchy

Hospital

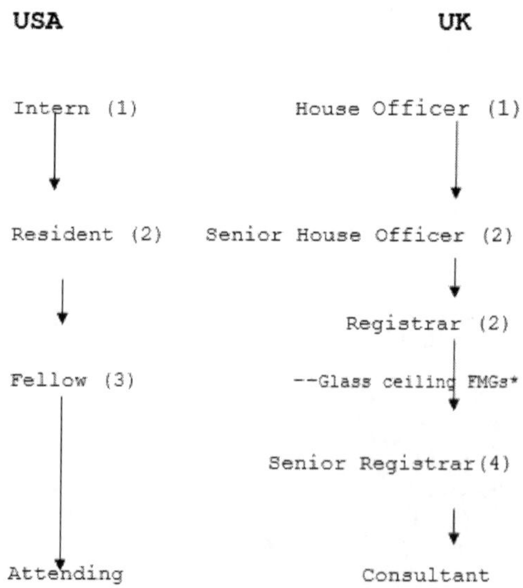

*Foreign Medical Graduates
( ) No. of years.

Fig 2. The Physician Hierarchy

Part One

The Itinerant Phase

CHAPTER ONE

The Beginning

I stood there for God knows how long, transfixed and completely overwhelmed by the sight: multiple escalators gliding upwards and downwards all around, and me, standing paralyzed in the middle. I felt like a village bumpkin who comes to a city for the first time.

With classical Indian music playing in the background, the Air India flight from Bombay stuttered and ground to a rough halt at its designated gate in London's Heathrow airport. It was July 18, 1980, a day that is still indelibly etched in my mind. I peered out of the tiny rectangular window to survey the landscape outside: my first glimpse of a foreign land, of Great Britain, of a country that I thought I knew so much about; yet I would realize soon how little I really knew.

The scene outside was uninviting: the sky was overcast with dark, heavy cumulus clouds that blanked out the sun's rays; visibility was hampered by dense gray smog, and droplets of water pattering on to the black, shiny tarmac made the ground look slippery and uncertain. Was the scene outside reflective of my days to come, I wondered.

The decision to come to the UK en route to a possible final destination of the US had not been easy. I had given up a much-sought-after postgraduate slot in a prestigious medical school in India to pursue this uncertain career path. The proverb a bird in hand is worth two in the bush had been quoted at me *ad nauseam*by my family, my mentor and my close friends. But overriding all opposition, I had embarked on this gamble. The stakes were high. Failure was not an option.

As I sat put in my seat staring out of the window and waiting for the seat belt sign to go off, a host of questions and doomsday scenarios swirled through my mind. What if I stumbled at the very first hurdle that I had to overcome, the PLAB exam? It would mean the end of my journey even before it started. I would have to return home having squandered a sum of money that would take me years to recoup. Such an outcome was not impossible. I had heard of students failing the exam despite two or three attempts.

Looming above all these queries was that million dollar question: Would I be eventually successful in reaching my final destination, the US? Or would I become another addition to the growing number of Indian physicians who had failed in their attempts to reach the US and been relegated to lifelong drudgery working in junior positions in dead-end gloomy,geriatric hospitals of the UK that offered little in terms of professional advancement?

I brushed aside these unnerving queries and tried to focus on my immediate priority: How do I reach Doncaster, where my uncle lived? There was no one to receive me at the airport. What appears simple now posed a daunting ordeal then. I had never interacted with full-blooded

Englishmen before; I had never seen an underground train and didn't have a clue about automatic dispensing machines.

After completing the formalities imposed by the customs and immigration agencies, I made my way to the Underground station, stopping on the way to ask for directions. The first thing that struck me as I spoke to airport officials was the accent: it was a far cry from the perfect intonation that marked the speech of BBC personnel. I had spent months listening to daily broadcasts of the BBC to acclimatize myself to what I had expected to encounter in this bastion of the English language. But what I now heard was a strange lingo that appeared to be English, yet was not English. I had to strain my ears and marshal my mental faculties to understand this garbled speech.

Later, I would learn that this was the famed Cockney accent that is prevalent in East London and is the lingua franca of the London working class. It is a sing-song incantation in which house becomes "ouse" and hair becomes "air". "Me" replaces "I" and words ending in "er" like dinner are pronounced as "dinna", an "a" replacing the "er". The end product is a distinctive dialect that an alien finds hard to comprehend.

I had waited barely a few minutes on the spotlessly clean, well-lit platform when a sleek, silver –colored train promptly arrived, a sharp contrast to the perpetual tardiness of trains in India of that time. Clumsily lugging my suitcase behind me, I clambered on to the train eyeing the automatic sliding doors with fascination and trepidation. Trains in India had manual doors or no doors at all and all this was new to me.

I found a vacant window seat and made myself comfortable. The inside of the train was immaculately clean by Indian standards and the blue cushioned seats were a step up in luxury compared to the hard wooden benches that graced the compartments of even long-distance trains back home. The commuters on the train presented a picture of discipline that I was not used to: an orderliness that was a far cry from the suffocating, overcrowded and disorderly scene common in Indian trains. The men, I noticed, were smartly suited: most of them wore ties and the light bounced off their black shiny shoes. And as for the women, they were almost picture perfect, clad in neatly pressed two-piece business suits or chic dress clothes. They sat straight-backed and staid-faced, some immersed in perusing the *Times*and others gazing ahead placidly. The silence that reigned despite the crowd was impressive.

The train traveled underground for a few miles before it surfaced to ground level, giving me my first glimpse of London and the UK. What I saw was a complete antithesis of my expectations. Rows of what I would come to know as “council homes” lined the streets on either side. Drab and archaic, these were dilapidated boxy edifices that were stuck together with barely any free space between each dwelling; not a pretty sight. The dirty ochre stain of their exterior walls, the broken windows and the sagging gray roofs made an already depressing sight even gloomier. The roads were certainly not paved with gold! I gaped in dismay and disbelief, where was the Britain I had heard so much about?

My immediate destination was a stop with a regal slant to its name and one that I had committed to memory, King’s Cross. I had to switch trains here to reach Doncaster in Yorkshire, my final destination.

King’s Cross/St Pancras is the biggest interchange station on the London Underground, with multiple commuter tracks crisscrossing at this point. It is also a major railway terminus that connects London with cities in the north and east of the UK, such as Cambridge, Hull, Doncaster, Leeds, Newcastle, Edinburgh and Glasgow.

As I picked my way through this bustling junction, I paused at the foot of an escalator bank for a brief respite; my hands were aching from the strain of carrying an unwieldy, awkward and heavy suitcase. Pull-on luggage was still unheard of at that time, or confined to those Indians who could boast of a relative or two in foreign countries.

That image and that moment at King's Cross has never left my mind.I stood there for God knows how long, transfixed and completely overwhelmed by the sight: multiple escalators gliding upwards and downwards all around, and me, standing paralyzed in the middle. I felt like a village bumpkin who comes to a city for the first time. The only escalator that I had come across so far was in a cinema hall in Bangalore (my hometown) where it had been installed more for show than out of necessity and made functional only on special occasions.

After a brief moment of cataplexy and a few queries, I gathered myself together, stepped onto the right escalator and managed to find the train to Doncaster.

It was Friday evening and the compartment was jam-packed with sweaty, pot-bellied men engaged in loud conversation with each other, most of them holding a bottle of beer in their hands. There didn't appear to be a ban on drinking in public places then. Looking back, I realize that the passengers were probably going to or coming from a football match. This crowd was distinctly different from the London crowd that I had encountered on the Underground; they appeared less sophisticated and less well-dressed. Unshaven beards, ill-fitting tee shirts and frayed jeans suggested a blue-collar background. Cigarette smoke diffused through the air making the whole scene hazy and mildly suffocating. I pushed myself into the compartment and located a convenient standing place; all seats had been taken and there was only standing room available.

I stood there amongst this motley crowd feeling no apprehension, no hint of fear of interacting with this football crowd. Were I to be placed in such a situation a few months later, I would have panicked and broken out into a cold sweat.

British football crowds are known for their uncouth behavior. Football hooliganism is almost a tradition in Britain with violent brawls breaking out routinely between supporters of rival teams during football matches. The first instances of football hooliganism date back to the late 1800s. This unruly tendency reached disturbing levels in the 70s and 80s. One notable incident that comes to mind is the Heysel Stadium Disaster. On May 29, 1985 prior to the start of the 1985 European Cup Finalbetween Liverpool of England and Juventus of Italy, a deadly melee broke out at the Heysel Stadium in Brussels, resulting in the death of 39 Juventus fans; another 600 were injured. An investigation into the disturbance concluded that English fans were totally responsible for the disaster, leading to a ban on English football teams and their fans from participating in European competitions for a protracted period of time.

Nearly 30 years later, there has been little change in the attitude of the British football hooligan. On March 17, 2013, Indian-origin football fan Prakash Patel, who had been returning home with his 21-year-old daughter after watching a Manchester United football game was mercilessly beaten up aboard a train after he objected to indecent racist remarks. What was even more shocking was that the 200-odd other passengers in the train failed to come to his help and in fact vied with one another to get a better 'ringside' view of the bashing.

The train ride was smooth and comfortable with none of the jolting and lurching that one commonly associated with Indian train journeys. About an hour and a half later, after racing past stations like Peterborough, Grantham and Newark, the train pulled into Doncaster. My uncle and his family with whom I was supposed to stay were away on a vacation in Europe but had kindly arranged for me to be picked up at the station by my aunt's nephew who happened to be working in Doncaster at that time. As soon as we reached my uncle's place, I threw myself on the bed. Exhausted by the whole experience, the long plane journey, the train ride and the new surroundings, I slept soundly and woke up 14 hours later, disturbed from my reverie by a mechanical purring sound that I couldn't quite place.........

CHAPTER TWO

You don't Make a Telegram.......

For a moment, there was dead silence at the other end. Then a cold female voice sternly admonished me, "You don't make a telegram, you send one!"

The purring sound continued, forcing me to pull myself out of bed and peek out of the bedroom window. It was the sound of a lawn mower. I could see a middle-aged man clad in shorts and a T-shirt busily working on his lawn, a tidy green piece of land that was pleasing to the eye and a far cry from the scraggly flora that passed for home gardens back in Bangalore, my hometown. I couldn't recall having seen a lawn mower till then. Both lawns and lawn mowers were uncommon in India and a novelty to me, like many other things I would come across in my early days in Britain.

Doncaster is a mid-sized city in the heart of Yorkshire County, approximately 30 kilometers from Sheffield. Among the flurry of new and strange-sounding names that assailed me in my early days, Yorkshire was one name I was familiar with, thanks to my interest in cricket.

Yorkshire, in my mind, was inseparably associated with Geoff Boycott, the stodgy but dependable English opener who had been a permanent member of the English cricket team for eons, from 1964 to 1982 to be exact. He was notorious for his slow run rate and extraordinary caution. Obsessed with not getting out, he played safe to the point of being boring and went for excruciatingly long periods without scoring any runs. It was his ability to remain grounded at the crease that earned him the distinction of being the only player in cricketing history to have batted on all 5 days of a test match, a feat that has never been replicated.

Yorkshire, located in the northeastern part of the country, is the largest county in England and covers an area close to 780 square miles. Important cities in Yorkshire include Leeds, a modern financial hub, and Sheffield, an industrial city known in the past for coal mining and steel plants. Doncaster, by contrast, was a low-key, non-descript second-tier city.

Nevertheless, even here in a second-tier city, everything I saw was an improvement over what we had in India. Roads were immaculately tarred and bereft of cumbersome bumps; potholes were almost non-existent. Spotlessly clean sidewalks separated roads from green manicured lawns and made the whole scene picture-perfect. This idyll was closer to the image of the UK that I had carried in my mind than the dismal scene I had encountered in London soon after landing at Heathrow airport.

Houses here were unlike their counterparts in India. Exterior walls did not sport the dull lime of plaster paint so typical of Indian houses. Houses had brick outer shells that were esthetically appealing despite not being painted over. Some houses had wood or vinyl sidings, something I had never seen before. Houses in India were all mortar and cement.

Moreover each of these dwellings was shaped differently from the others, quite a change from the uniformity of the boxy models of urban India. And the roofs were not flat but tangentially sloped, another variation that I gathered was intended to keep snow from accumulating in winter. The interior too was dissimilar. Floors were covered with carpet from one wall to another, a distinct change from India where floors rarely had carpets and bare red copper oxide floors were the invariable norm.

Additionally, homes here had air conditioning and heating which kept the internal environment pleasant despite the vagaries of the weather outside. The air was pure and household furniture barely collected any dust or dirt, yet another contrast from India, where homes had to be cleaned twice a day to keep the dust from accumulating.

Faucets dispensing cold and hot water were a welcome novelty to me and so was the copious and continuous supply of water. I could take a bath at any time of the day without an elaborate preparation or wait. Electric water heaters in bathrooms were still a luxury in the India of the 1980s, being restricted to the homes of the well-off; apart from being dangerous, these heaters had to be activated by a switch that had to be turned on at least 30 minutes prior to one's bath.

Most Indian bathrooms then got by with a primitive hot water boiler system, an elaborate structure that consisted of a large copper cauldron embedded in a rectangular cake of cement with an opening at the bottom that accepted coal, wood or cow dung cakes (patties of dried cow dung) as fuel. Each morning, the water heating process had to be initiated manually, a ritual that involved placing a stack of cow dung cakes under the cauldron, dousing them with kerosene oil and striking a match to get the fire going. This exercise would be repeated religiously and uncertainly every day, followed by constant supervision to ensure that the fire did not die out. Otherwise, one could return an hour later to face an urn full of cold water and the prospect of a chilly bath.

Local transport in Doncaster was cheap. The fare for any ride was a mere two pence. Yellow-colored double-decker buses were plentiful and ran on time. One hardly had to wait for a few minutes before another bus arrived. Space was never a problem and for the most part buses ran empty or near empty.

I noticed that bus drivers here doubled as ticket dispensers as well, unlike the Indian system where two persons manned every bus, one to drive the bus and another, the "conductor", to collect fares. It was my interaction with bus drivers which first alerted me to the nuances of the Yorkshire accent.

The "u" sound is pronounced as "oo" so that "up" becomes "oop" and "cup" becomes "coop." There is a distinct drawl attached to words that have an "a" sound in the middle of a word with words like "care" being enunciated as "caare." Words that end in "ake" are shortened to sound like "ek." Take becomes "tek" and "make" becomes "mek." All these peculiarities make the sing-song Yorkshire accent quite different from the Queen's English and it takes some time to get accustomed to it. However within a few days I found myself unconsciously conversing in the local lingo.

While the modern amenities that I encountered impressed me, one thought troubled my mind. If Britain was a benign colonial power as claimed by its apologists, why did these two countries, India and Britain, demonstrate such stark differences in basic amenities? All this progress in Britain had not occurred in the last 30 years after its fracture from India: it must have taken longer than that. Britain and India had been under the same administration for over 200 years; yet when the British left India in 1947 India was a hapless Third World nation with people lacking even basic facilities like running water and electricity. All this only affirmed my belief that there is no such thing as "good colonialism." It was a myth propagated by ex-colonial powers as a face-saving ploy to conform to changing times and assuage the guilt they felt.

George Monbiot, an English writer for *The Guardian*confirms my assessment and provides an overview of the fiscal and social consequences of British colonialism in India in one his columns. He writes:

> "*For the past 300 years, the revolutions and reforms experienced by almost all other developed countries have been averted in Britain by foreign remittances.*
>
> *The social unrest which might have transformed our politics was instead outsourced to our colonies and unwilling trading partners. The rebellions in Ireland, India, China, the Caribbean, Egypt, South Africa, Malaya, Kenya, Iran and other*

> *places we subjugated were the price of political peace in Britain...*
>
> *There will probably never be a full account of the robbery this country organised, but there are a few snapshots. In his book Capitalism and Colonial Production, Hamza Alavi estimates that the resource flow from India to Britain between 1793 and 1803 was in the order of £2m a year, the equivalent of many billions today. The economic drain from India, he notes, "has not only been a major factor in India's impoverishment...it has also been a very significant factor in the Industrial Revolution in Britain." As Ralph Davis observes in The Industrial Revolution and British Overseas Trade, from the 1760s onwards India's wealth "bought the national debt back from the Dutch and others...leaving Britain nearly free from overseas indebtedness when it came to face the great French wars from 1793."*

The human cost of this financial exploitation was enormous and callous. Monbiot elaborates:

> *"Just as grain was sucked out of Ireland at the height of its great famine, so Britain continued to drain India of food during its catastrophic hungers. In Late Victorian Holocausts, Mike Davis shows that Indian wheat exports to the UK doubled between 1876 and 1877 as subsistence there collapsed. Several million Indians died of starvation. In the North-Western provinces the famine was wholly engineered by British policy, as their surplus production was exported to offset poor*

English harvests in 1876 and 1877..

In the late 19th Century, Davis shows, Britain's vast deficits with the United States, Germany and its white Dominions were balanced by huge annual surpluses with India and (as a result of the opium trade) China. .....Britain's trade surpluses with India allowed the City to become the world's financial capital.

The great British adventure – three centuries spent pillaging the labour, wealth and resources of other countries – is over."

("Outsourcing Unrest," The Guardian, June 9, 2009)

With such large-scale plunder stretching out over three centuries, India's consequent penury was certain and its pathetic plight at the time of its independence understandable. But a poor man is rarely asked an explanation for his poverty. He is judged on his appearance and so was the case with India in the period from 1947 to the early 1990s.

This opening paragraph from Alex Tunzelmann's book, *Indian Summer: The Secret History of the End of an Empire*, aptly reflects the reversal of fortunes that colonialism effected. Describing the scene in pre-colonial times she writes:

"*In the beginning there were two nations. One was a vast, mighty and magnificent empire, brilliantly organized and culturally unified, which dominated a massive swath of the earth. The other was an undeveloped semi-feudal realm, riven by religious factionalism and barely able to feed its illiterate, diseased and stinking masses. The first nation was India. The second was England.*"

By 1947 when the British had finished with India the transposition was complete: affluent India had become poor and indigent England rich.

Doncaster was also the place where I had my first experience of British snobbery. A telephone call from the UK to India was a cumbersome venture involving a telephone operator, advance booking and poor connections that crackled with static, making the faint voice that emanated from the telephone even more incomprehensible. Moreover it was expensive. So I decided to send a telegram to intimate my folks in India of my safe arrival. Sending a telegram was quite easy here: no trek to the post office, no long lines or officious forms to fill out. One could pick up a phone and get the job done.

During my initial days, I was apprehensive of interacting with locals even over the phone. In my nervousness I blurted out, "Can I make a telegram?" For a moment, there was dead silence at the other end. Then a cold female voice sternly admonished me, "You don't *make*a telegram, you *send* one!"

CHAPTER THREE

LONDON, YMCA AND A £2 NAN

Taking a cue from the saying, "See Naples and die," I urged myself to "See London and go home."

The building had a non-descript exterior, a brick front that opened out onto the street below through an unimpressive faded wooden door. Nevertheless it was a haven for students from India like me. It was the Indian YMCA in London, a place that would become a frequent haunt of mine in the coming months and years. And it was here that I stayed when I returned to London to appear for the PLAB exam, approximately two weeks after I had landed at Heathrow airport.

The YMCA is conveniently located in the heart of London in Fitzroy Square and is within walking distance of the Warren Street Tube station, making it easy to locate and to access for new migrants from India.

The Indian YMCA is unlike other YMCAs: it has a distinct Indian flavor and a history of its own. Despite several transformations and translocations, it has maintained its unique place among the Indian community here. It was founded in 1920 by the National Council of the YMCA of India and has been a place of refuge for scores of Indian students fresh off the boat. In its early days, I was told, the YMCA functioned out of an ad hoc structure near London University before moving to a permanent site at Gower Street in 1923.

Gower Street remained the home of the YMCA for close to 20 years before the building was partially wrecked by a German bomb in World War II. During this period, the YMCA became a hub of Indian nationalistic activity, hosting debates and discussions that saw the likes of Netaji Subhas Chandra Bose, Lala Lajpat Rai, Sarojini Naidu, Acharya J. B. Kripalani and Jayaprakash Narayan, all famous Indian freedom fighters, come through its doors. Even Mahatma Gandhi visited this place in 1931 to conduct an inter-faith dialog.

The present edifice, constructed in 1953, has undergone extensive renovations and extensions, with the last one being in 2004. While the YMCA does promote a spectrum of activities that are educational, social and cultural in nature, it is mostly popular for the accommodation that it provides: both daily and long-term stays are entertained.

Evening shadows were lengthening when I reached the YMCA. It was past 7 PM. The cafeteria was closed and the receptionist, a young, friendly part-time student, directed me to an Indian restaurant a block away. They make a good

*Malai Kofta,*he had advised. The restaurant called Indian Taj was a modest place, dimly lit as most restaurants are, and practically empty. In fact, I was the only customer that evening. A strong scent of curry filled the air and made me feel at home. But as I leafed through the dog-eared menu, I was in for a surprise. For a moment I couldn't believe my eyes. The cost of one *nan* (Indian flatbread) was an incredible two pounds.

The price, if I recollect rightly, did include a vegetable entrée; but even that failed to temper the sticker shock. A quick mental calculation only added to my discomfort. Two pounds translated to 40 Indian rupees then, a princely sum in those days. I could easily have had 10 meals for that amount back home. I just couldn't bring myself to cough up 40 rupees for something that could be bought in India for one or two rupees, at the most. But I was starving and had to eat something, perforce. Conscious of my limited resources - I had barely 50 pounds in my pocket which had to cover my entire London trip - I grudgingly ordered a single piece of nan and a vegetable curry to go with it. I ate my meal slowly, making sure that I savored every bit of this pricey nan.

When I had finished my meal and was preparing to leave, one of the waiters approached me and asked politely: "Sir, would you like me to pack the leftovers?'

I was taken aback and responded with a look of affront and puzzlement. Indignantly I shook my head, controlled myself from retorting angrily, paid the bill and walked out of the restaurant. Packing up leftovers was not a custom that was common in India. Moreover it was considered to be the act of a cheapskate.

Compared to this sparse and expensive meal, the lunch that I had the following day in the YMCA cafeteria was a gourmet serving replete with two types of curried vegetables, hot piping sambhar(South Indian lentil soup), rice and roti (flat unleavened Indian bread). There was even a fried golden pappadam (crisp) and a slice of lemon pickle to go with it, all for one pound. This was a meal I would enjoy again and again, making it a point to visit the YMCA whenever I happened to be in the vicinity of London.

The accommodation at the YMCA was spartan. The room was no more than a cubbyhole but enough to serve one's needs. There were only two pieces of furniture in the room: a small bed covered with striped sheets that were more reminiscent of India than Britain, and a compact writing desk. There was no clock or telephone. However the tariff, Indianism for room rates and a term that the YMCA continued to use even in London, was a modest eight pounds, a feature that made the accommodation additionally attractive.

The PLAB exam was an experience in itself. The topical content was manageable. It was the English language section that proved to be challenging: an exercise in audio comprehension, it consisted of 15 to 20 recorded conversation pieces representative of Britain's various accents that were played back in quick succession for us candidates to transcribe into plain English. Attempting to decipher the garbled speech became an even more formidable task in the tense atmosphere of the exam hall and in the limited time frame. I could barely comprehend half of the sentences. I came out of the exam hall, certain that I had flunked this section.

That evening, in the throes of post-exam blues, I speculated on the outcome of the exam and my future. What if I failed the exam? What would I do? What a colossal waste of money! Would I have to go back to India, never to return to the West again? After mulling over these despondent questions for some time, I pulled myself together. Forget the future I told myself. Savor the moment. You are in London, one of the great cities of the world. Go out and take in the sights of this historic city. Taking a cue from the saying, "See Naples and die," I urged myself to "See London and go home."

So that is what I did. I hopped on to one of those red double-decker sight-seeing buses and went on a jaunt of London. The trip had a two-hour itinerary that took us past Buckingham Palace, the Tower of London, London Bridge and Big Ben. The structures were imposing but in my dejected frame of mind, I really could not enjoy their beauty. I felt like a robot going through the motions.

The next day I returned to Doncaster to await my results: three long weeks that seemed to stretch interminably before me.

CHAPTER FOUR

WAITING FOR THE RESULTS

Did the size of the envelope mean the presence of re-application forms for another attempt- a sign of failure?

Waiting for anything is an unpleasant experience, but when it is for the results of an exam on which hinges the future course of your career, it can be particularly painful and nerve-wracking.

Mellowed by age, today I have a different perspective, a more comprehensive view of life. But as a young adult, my mind was obsessed with achieving professional success. In my 20s, I subscribed to this lop-sided notion that apportioned 80 percent of life's success to the achievement of professional goals. Every step therefore appeared crucial, every career-related event carried with it a make-or-break potential: something like a game of snakes and ladders in which one slip could bring you tumbling down to the starting block.

By the time I returned from London to Doncaster, my uncle's family had returned from their trip abroad. Kitukaka (Kitu being a short form of Krishna and *kaka*meaning uncle) as I called him was really not my uncle. He was my mother's uncle. Interestingly, he was only 2 years older than my mother, being the ninth of my great grandfather's ten children.

Kitukaka was also a physician and had spent over 20 years practicing medicine in Belgaum, a moderately large town in the southern Indian state of Karnataka, whose capital, Bengaluru (earlier Bangalore) is now a famous IT hub. In the mid-70s, he had suddenly decided to wrap up his practice and move to the UK. Here, he had quickly settled down as a general practitioner without much difficulty. Kitukaka and his family would be a great source of mental and physical strength to me during my stay in the UK. They were there for me whenever I needed any help, financial or emotional.

I spent "the waiting period" reading books, watching TV and trying to make myself helpful around the house. Kids here, I noted, were a part of the home workforce obligated to "do the dishes" and wash the laundry albeit with the help of modern technology in the form of washers and dryers. I tried my best to lend a helping hand in these daily chores, but was kept away since making a guest do the dishes was considered bad hospitality.

This forced respite also gave me an opportunity to interact with many of my uncle's friends who dropped in on the weekends. Most of them were general practitioners like him and hailed from either Karnataka or its neighboring state, Maharashtra. These get-togethers gave me a glimpse of the contrasting nouveau immigrant attitudes prevailing in the community as exemplified by two frequent visitors to my uncle's home.

Dr Kumar was a balding man in his early 40s whose conversation invariably hovered around his travails at his workplace which he perceived to be discriminatory in nature. He was an experienced physician who had graduated from a good medical school in India at least 15 years prior. But now he was stuck in a dead-end career track that involved shifting base every six months and working at a trainee level suited for someone barely out of medical school. Pathos poured out of him as he reiterated his crushed ambition of becoming a neurologist and narrated to us the daily humiliation that he suffered from less qualified junior doctors who lorded over him simply because they were British.

Countering this view was a distinguished elderly academic, Dr Ramesh, who was a lecturer in statistics at Birmingham University. He was not a doctor of medicine but a PhD, and appeared to have done well in his professional career. He contended much to the consternation of the others that it was intellectual mediocrity of people like Kumar (although he didn't specifically mention him by name) that pushed them to use racism as a scapegoat to cover up their shortcomings. And so the arguments continued, sometimes late into the night, punctuated by breaks for dinner and repeated interruptions by the ladies who exhorted them to switch to more pleasant topics.

Lost in these polemics, I was able to overcome, at least temporarily, my anxiety as I waited for my exam results. During those tense days I even contemplated going to neighboring Ireland in search of a job. Ireland, unlike the UK, shared reciprocity with India enabling Indian physicians to practice in Ireland without the hassle of a qualifying exam. But scant job opportunities made the task of obtaining a job there much more difficult than in the UK.

Finally one Thursday afternoon the moment of reckoning arrived when the shuffling sound of mail being slipped underneath the door brought me rushing to the main entrance (a daily ritual that I had followed for the preceding three weeks). Lying on the carpet was a large brown envelope bearing the stamp of the General Medical Council. My heart was beating faster, my palms were moist with sweat and conflicting thoughts raced through my mind. Did the size of the envelope mean the presence of re-application forms for another attempt- a sign of failure? I stood transfixed for a moment. Then with a prayer on my lips, I tore open the envelope. I had passed. I felt more relieved than happy as I slumped onto the living room sofa reading the letter over and over again to confirm my success.

Without wasting any time, I began in earnest the next phase of my overseas adventure, looking for a job – or a "locum" job to be more precise.

I had been warned that finding a "permanent job", as opposed to a locum, was impossible in the initial stages. Permanency, I learnt was a relative term in reference to the career of a junior immigrant doctor in the UK. The normal duration of a "permanent job" for a junior doctor was a mere six months that could be stretched out to one year and a half at the discretion of the authorities. If a permanent position lasted only six months, a locum perforce had to be shorter in duration. The shortest locum that I was called upon to do lasted a mere two days. Most locum durations however could be counted in weeks. Rarely could one find a position that required your services for a month or two.

Locums were necessary to fill vacancies created by physicians on leave. Junior doctors in the UK are strongly bonded into a union that fiercely protects their interests, and the union is not averse to using strong-arm tactics like strikes to get its way. The presence of a powerful union acted like a buffer and prevented doctors from being overworked when their colleagues vacationed; hence the concept of locums.

It was easy to land a locum position as it was a temporary arrangement and did not call for extensive scrutiny; all that the authorities needed was a warm body to promptly fill the vacuum. Decisions had to be made quickly and frequently, and deals were sealed via a phone interview without the formal face-to-face meeting.

Timing however was key: one had to be the first to contact the hospital once a vacancy became available. This resulted in a mad rush to get one's hands on the *British Medical Journal* (or *BMJ* as it was popularly known) that came out once a week and was a repository of notifications about locums as well as "permanent jobs." But, as I soon discovered, a week could be a long time in this rat race. One had to be proactive and call the British Medical Association (BMA) locum agency every morning and evening, which I did, for possible new leads. The locum agency updated its list of job opportunities every day and many openings were usually filled by the time they appeared in the print edition that came out later in the week.

The career path for junior doctors in the UK, as I look back on it today, strikes me as being unorganized and haphazard. There were four different levels of training, starting with the position of a house officer meant for physicians fresh out of medical school. After a six-month to one-year stint as a house officer, one progressed to become a senior house officer or SHO. The next level was that of a registrar. Technically one could advance to a registrar position after training as an SHO for one year. But that was never the case with immigrant doctors especially those from the subcontinent. I found senior physicians from India, Pakistan and Sri Lanka languishing as SHOs for years together and some, unfortunately, spent their entire career at this grade.

The barrier to becoming a registrar was a hurdle that could be breached with some persistence. However, it was the next step in the ladder that reached the impenetrable glass ceiling. Experience as a senior registrar, the last training grade, was a prerequisite for becoming a consultant. Senior registrar positions were available only at major hospitals located in urban medical centers and were, for all intents and purposes off limits to "foreigners." A senior registrar usually served out a four-year term.

The most unsettling aspect of the training of junior doctors in the UK was its uncertainty. There was no orderly transition from one level to another as in the American system where an intern (equivalent to a house officer) automatically moves up to become a second-year resident and then a third-year resident upon satisfactory completion of each year of training. In the UK, each position was a separate entity that had to be sought and attained *de novo*. Promotion to a higher grade was not guaranteed even after satisfactorily completing the lower grade. This invariably led to stagnation mostly at the SHO stage for many an Indian doctor.

The consultant's position, which many foreign doctors aspired to reach but never did, was the pinnacle of the NHS physician hierarchy. When some foreign doctors did manage to overcome by some act of providence the insurmountable difficulties that came their way, and did fulfill the requirements needed to become a consultant, they were assigned to specialties like geriatrics (care of the elderly) that local graduates cared little for. In fact, I came across a fair number of Indian, Pakistani and Bangladeshi consultants in geriatrics during my travels across the UK.

As opposed to the temporary nature of training positions, a consultant post was a permanent job: so permanent was its nature that it was jokingly said that no one except Her Royal Highness, the Queen of Britain possessed the authority to relieve a consultant of his/her duties. This permanency imbued many a consultant with a sense of arrogance and made them indulge in excesses that would not have been normally tolerated. There were anecdotes of a consultant who regularly guided ward rounds from the comfort of his sailboat on the lake. This could have been an exaggeration, but stories about consultants sneaking away to take in a game of golf during the course of the day, especially in the summer, were well known.

After sending out innumerable copies of my résumé every week for almost a month, most of which remained unacknowledged or were responded to with a standard letter of rejection, I finally got a break through the BMA agency. However, there was a catch.

CHAPTER FIVE

MONIKERS AND A TASTE OF ENGLISH FOOD

To this, Dr Krishnamachari politely replied that it would be acceptable as long as he too had the license to address Dr Thomas Rogers as "Tiruchirapalli Rajagopalachari"

"They need a locum in geriatrics at St. Margaret's Hospital in Epping. An SHO is going on leave for an extended period of 6 weeks and they want someone who can start the day after tomorrow. You had better call them now." The lady from the BMA office told me.

But I hesitated. I had some misgivings about accepting a position in geriatrics, which was considered an unglamorous and dull branch of medicine. Moreover, I had heard that once you started working in geriatrics, your chances of getting a position in general medicine, in which

I was interested, dropped considerably. But after having drawn a blank for over a month and with my monetary resources dwindling, I realized that I could not afford to be choosy. I decided to explore the option.

I dialed the hospital and spoke to the consultant in charge, Dr. Roy, who spoke to me for no more than a minute, offered me the job and hung up.

There was a small formality to be completed before I began my job. I had to journey to Croydon, located in the south of England, to obtain a work permit issued by the Home Office. Unlike the process of obtaining a work permit in the US, which can be a cumbersome, expensive and lengthy legal matter, the process here was hassle-free. A work permit could be obtained on the spot by walking into the concerned office. All that was required was a nominal job offer; even a locum position was acceptable for this purpose. Armed with the stamp of approval that allowed me 'leave of stay' for a period of one year, till September 14, 1981, I set out to begin my first job in the UK.

Epping was a small town more famous for the forest that goes by its name than for the town itself, and was located about 15 miles to the northeast of London. It was, for all intents and purposes, a suburb of London. The town was well connected to the city by the London Underground (subway) and was the eastern terminus of the Central Line.

Dusk was setting in when I was dropped off at St Margaret's Hospital by one of those iconic bumblebee-shaped black London cabs that I had hired at the Tube station. St Margaret's Hospital was a grim collection of motley buildings spread out over a large ground encircled by a dense forest of trees that formed a natural boundary around the hospital enclave. There was no designated reception area or a formal entrance. I looked around and found a helpful passer-by who guided me to the hospital ward that I was supposed to report to.

The first person that I encountered there was Sister Green, the head nurse of the ward. Nurses in the UK, as in India, are traditionally addressed as "Sister." Strictly speaking, "sister" is a prefix that is applicable only to a head nurse; however it has come to be used as a generic term to address all nurses. But God forbid if you employ this honorific to beckon a nurse in the US. A friend of mine recounted an embarrassing incident in which he was curtly told by a nurse that she was not his "sister."

Head nurses in the UK constitute a breed by themselves and it was rumored that one had to belong to the pedigreed class to aspire to a head nurse position, especially in the more prestigious hospitals. Stern and matronly, these worthies rule over their turf with an iron hand and a no-nonsense demeanor that make young house officers quake with trepidation and student nurses cry. Even consultants are hard put to overrule their concerns, and seek their counsel when evaluating junior doctors.

Sister Green was slightly more humane and less snobbish than the other "Sisters" that I would work with during my stay in the UK. She was a well-built woman, handsome in her own way, with a chubby friendly face. Her smile revealed just a hint of condescension as she welcomed me to the unit and bade me to wait at the nurses' station. She informed me that Dr Marion, my registrar, would soon be there to take me around, and proceeded to fill me in on Dr Marion, telling me how nice and efficient he was.

As I waited for Dr Marion to arrive, I conjured up an image of a white Anglo-Saxon physician with a clipped

English accent. So I was a little taken aback when in walked a dark-complexioned gentleman of medium height clad in a long white coat that fell below his knees. He greeted me with a heavily accented "hello" that did not have the intonation of the Queen's English. As he continued to speak, I noticed that his English had a peculiar sing-song manner that I would soon learn was characteristic of people from Sri Lanka – or Ceylon as it was called earlier.

Dr Marion was in reality Dr Marianyagam, a physician from the island of Sri Lanka, whose name had been cut short to make it easy on the tongues of local British folk. It is a common practice in the UK to exchange foreign names for British monikers, a practice that is practically expedient, but one that also denotes insensitivity to a foreigner's identity.

In this context, I am compelled to recount an interesting banter that supposedly occurred between a certain Dr Tiruchirapalli Krishnamachari from Chennai, India, and a Dr Thomas Rogers from Birmingham. Overwhelmed by this 28-letter south Indian tongue-twister, Dr Rogers, the consultant queried Dr Krishnamachari whether he was okay with the moniker of 'Chris'. To this, Dr Krishnamachari politely replied that it would be acceptable as long as he too had the license to address Dr Thomas Rogers as "Tiruchirapalli Rajagopalachari". Dr Rogers took the hint, dropped the idea and made a serious attempt to carefully pronounce the name "Krishnamachari" from that moment onwards.

Dr Marion was an affable, easy-going person who was of great help to me as I tried to understand and carry out my expected duties in this new environment. To be honest, working in a geriatric ward is not a challenging experience from a professional standpoint. I was not excited to be there. There were no patients that required acute medical care and no emergencies that required prompt attention.

However, some of my preconceived notion about geriatrics proved to be wrong. There were redeeming facets to this medical specialty that made it interesting. Diseases in the elderly manifest themselves with subtle symptoms, in contrast to an overt presentation seen in younger adults. For example, the classic symptoms of pneumonia in a young patient are cough and fever, while this same disease manifests itself in an old man or woman as something as unrelated as mental confusion. Extensive detective work was necessary in many cases to decipher the cause of a problem, especially in those patients who were dysphasic as a result of strokes and thus unable to express themselves.

Nevertheless, I found the pace of work too slow for my likening. I was in charge of about 25 patients, all of whom were over 65 years of age and many of whom were bedridden. My daily routine involved making rounds with Dr Marianyagam and Sister Green. Rounds meant moving from patient to patient with a cart full of charts in which I dutifully recorded the daily status of each patient. Every patient was physically examined, his or her medication list was reviewed, and blood test results were checked for any abnormalities that needed correction. This ritual was repeated with each patient until we had exhausted the entire complement of the ward.

Dr Roy, our consultant, was a bespectacled kindly soul with a receding hairline and a soft, halting manner of speech. My guess was that he was in his early 60s as he often spoke of retirement. He had been in Britain for over 20 years, was content with what he had achieved in the course of his career and had no plans of returning to India. Monday afternoon and Friday mornings were the two days that he rounded with us, carefully supervising our work and ensuring that we did not make any obvious mistakes. But there was hardly any need for that. Dr Marion was an extremely competent registrar and there was very little that Dr Roy could add to his management style.

In fact, in most teaching hospitals - hospitals with trainee physicians - it is the registrars or senior registrars who "run the show." Consultants are for the most part bystanders jumping in occasionally with "editorial comments" made more to justify their existence than to effect any tangible change in the treatment.

Being "on call," the age-old tradition of being available for medical emergencies that occur after the end of a normal working day and before the next one begins, is an intrinsic part of a physician's job description. The "on call" period includes weekday nights and the weekend. The weekend may be split into Saturday and Sunday with the change of guard occurring after 24 hours, or it can be one continuous and arduous stretch extending from Friday evening to Monday morning. Weekend call in UK usually took the latter form and was something to be dreaded. While fully trained physicians also continue to take "on call" duties throughout their careers, resident doctors are at the forefront of this "war on emergencies" and take what is in medical jargon called "first call." I still recall the utter fear that used to grip me as Friday evening approached and the relief I felt when Monday morning arrived.

Back in India, I had been trained at one of the top medical schools in the country, JIPMER. JIPMER, an acronym for Jawaharlal Institute of Medical Education and Research, is a federally funded medical institute based in Pondicherry (now Puducherry) a Union Territory situated on the southeast coast of India just south of Chennai.

There we had a structured training system with multiple tiers of trainees being rostered for on call duty. An "on call" team comprised an intern, a junior resident (2 years post medical school) and a senior resident. All members of this team were actively involved in managing emergency medical care. However, here in the UK it was significantly different. There was either a house officer (intern) or senior house officer available on call, backed up by a registrar (senior resident), and the unwritten rule was that the house officer did not bother the registrar until something earth-shattering took place. This resulted in inexperienced overworked house officers making medical decisions that were clearly beyond their level of training, guided by nothing more than the concise emergency manual that they carried around and referred to faithfully.

A rather disturbing medical anecdote was making the rounds in my early days in Epping. It concerned a recently graduated house officer from a nearby hospital. Around midnight one day he had been called to attend to a patient in the emergency room. The patient, a 65-year-old gentleman had come in with palpitations and had been found to be in acute atrial fibrillation, a disturbance of the heart rhythm that can be fatal if not treated promptly. After examining the patient, our young doctor, brimming with the confidence that only a greenhorn can possess, had promptly looked up the treatment of atrial fibrillation prescribed in his little book and proceeded to inject the patient with a dose of amiodarone, a medication that had just come on the market. The consequences were disastrous. The patient went into cardiac arrest and died immediately.

The medical fraternity can be scathing in its criticism in the face of adverse events and the local group of physicians was no different. Rumors ran rife. Some claimed that the house officer had pushed in the medication too rapidly instead of injecting it slowly over 10 minutes. Still others believed that the house officer had administered the medication without placing the patient on a monitor that displayed the heart rhythm in real time allowing for detection and correction of adverse events that can occur as a result of amiodarone. Whatever the truth, one thing was clear: the degree of supervision prevalent then in the UK was woefully inadequate.

My stay at Epping was an initiation for me on several fronts, food being one of them. After spending two months in the sheltered eating environment of my uncle's home where I was fed excellent home-made Indian food on a daily basis, I was not prepared for what I faced. In Epping, I felt as though I'd been thrown out into a culinary wilderness to face the raw insipidity of English cuisine. To make matters worse, I was a vegetarian – or rather, an eggetarian to be more precise.

The blandness of English food struck me on my very first day. Late in the evening when I walked into the cafeteria and asked for something that did not contain meat or fish, the server behind the counter placed two slices of bread, a small mound of cooked peas and a boiled potato on a plate and handed it to me. I tried to make this drab meal more palatable by adding a generous sprinkling of salt and pepper, but to no avail. Add to this the depressing locale: the room was empty, the light was dim and, it was wintry cold. An already tasteless meal became even more insipid. I just could not bring myself to force this food down my throat. After a bite or two I walked out of the cafeteria, my stomach still empty.

The next day I was able to go out and buy packets of powdered tomato soup which proved to be tastier than what I had encountered in the cafeteria the night before. The soup was easy to make. All I had to do was to dissolve the contents of the packet in hot water that was readily available at the sink in my room. This instant soup along with two slices of plain bread became the staple elements of my dinner for the next few days until I became more familiar with my new surroundings and was able to go out and find other palatable items.

In 2 weeks, I had settled into an acceptable routine at Epping. I was even beginning to like the place when I was jolted out of my comfort zone by a rude shock.

CHAPTER SIX

" YOU, DIRTY PAKI"

They encircled me; the hefty looking one with the tattoo on his arm stood directly in front of me while the other two flanked him on either side.

She was extremely old, archaic to be more descriptive. She was lying crumpled in her hospital bed, her extremities distorted and her fingers gnarled by rheumatoid arthritis. She must have been close to 90 years old. Her hair was disheveled and fell all over her wrinkled face. For a moment, I felt that she was dysphasic and incapable of expressing herself. Then the words flew across the room, a spittle of venom that threw me off balance.

"Blackie, blackie!" she screamed pointing to me and another physician, "I don't want to be treated by blackies."

All of us, the two foreign doctors and the English nurse who were making rounds that morning were dumbstruck.

An uncomfortable moment ensued with everyone present being too embarrassed to confront the issue. Then pretending that nothing of note had occurred, we moved on to the next patient.

That was my first brush with racism in Britain.

That particular incident did not disturb me greatly. But a few days later, I was to experience an ugly racial encounter that would leave an indelible imprint on my mind and profoundly affect my day-to-day behavior.

Weekends in Epping proved to be a bonanza. I had ample time to explore my surroundings for some eatables. I ventured into the local supermarket and spent hours together scouring the aisles for anything that even faintly resembled Indian food to make my meals more palatable. Those days were a far cry from the Britain of today, when one can walk into a grocery store and find shelves bursting with a variety of Indian foods ranging from condiments like chutneys to full-fledged gourmet meals that come in a variety of brands packaged in all sizes. The *Patak* brand, ubiquitous in recent times, was then confined to small pop-and-mom Indian outlets that graced street corners; with no car to travel around, I was oblivious to the existence of these shops in my early days.

It was during one of those long boring weekends and my continuing quest for good food that I rediscovered the Indian YMCA in London. Epping, as I mentioned earlier, was located on the outskirts of London, and could be accessed easily via the London Underground. The Central line extended all the way up to Epping and was extremely convenient.

This discovery made my weekends more exciting as I developed a set weekend routine. This involved traveling into London early in the morning, roaming its crowded streets till late in the afternoon, and finally capping it off with a sumptuous but inexpensive lunch at the YMCA.

Oxford Street was a favorite haunt of mine during these excursions. The bustling crowds reminded me of Indian streets and made me feel surprisingly comfortable. I spent hours together strolling aimlessly up and down the street gawking at window displays and occasionally dropping into a shop to explore its interior. I did little buying despite the fact that my initial paychecks brought in what I considered at that time to be a good amount. I thought it prudent to be frugal in light of my uncertain future.

On one of these London trips I even paid a visit to Harrods that proclaims itself as the largest department store in the world. Harrods is located in the Knightsbridge area, a few stops away from Oxford Circus. The store was expansive, spanning an area of 4.5 acres with a selling space of over a million square feet. I spent almost half a day exploring the grandeur of the store and the diversity of its contents.

These weekend jaunts were refreshing and relaxing. I was beginning to enjoy and like this new country.

The journey back and forth to London took approximately an hour, the Tube route meandering its way through parts of east London popularly known as the East End. On this line one came across stops with names like Bethnal Green and Mile End. It was obvious to me even as a newcomer to the country that this was an underprivileged part of London. The train stations bore a deserted, uncared for look. Historically, the East End has been a crowded place known for its poverty and immigrant population. Initially home to Irish immigrants, it later housed a large Bangladeshi community. The white population that lived here was traditionally working class and poor. The people getting on and off at these stops mirrored the socio-economic status of this area.

It happened one Saturday evening when I was returning from London. It had been a routine weekend outing for me, enjoyable and relaxing having spent the day doing my routine jig complete with the appetizing noon meal at the YMCA.I settled into my seat by the window on the train, opened up the newspaper that I had picked up earlier and began browsing through it, occasionally looking out of the window to take in the sights. At first everything seemed normal: passengers entering and getting off as the train halted at stops that had become familiar to me.

I think it was somewhere between Mile End and Bethnal Green (red line) when I noticed that the compartment was almost empty except for a gang of teenagers. There were four of them, three boys and a girl. Two of the boys sported black leather jackets, one full-sleeved and the other sleeveless, revealing a large tattoo covering the entire circumference of bulging right biceps. Both were wearing faded blue jeans splashed in parts with bleach that gave them a rugged look. The lower end of their jeans was tucked into heavy black boots that came almost up to their knees. The third boy appeared slightly younger and was clad in a checkered blue shirt and beige colored baggy trousers held up by a pair of red suspenders.

All the boys had close-cropped hair that made them look almost bald. I froze for a moment. These were skinheads.

Skinheads belonged to a subculture that took root among the working-class youth of Britain in the 1960s. The distinctive feature of these skinheads was their close-cropped hair style. It was a culture that was initially based on fashion, music and lifestyle, but which later on degenerated to include racist violence and right-wing politics. In the early 80s, skinheads became an important constituent of the British National Front, a right-wing political party that believed in white supremacy.

Paki-bashing was a term made popular by skinheads, the term 'Paki' being a generic one that included Indians, Pakistanis and Bangladeshis - that is, all brown-skinned folks. At first, there were isolated reports of individual skinheads waylaying immigrants, but soon Paki-bashing became a popular group pastime among skinheads. On Friday nights and Saturday afternoons, when town centers milled with shopping crowds, it was not uncommon to find gangs of drunken skinheads roaming the streets looking for unsuspecting Asian immigrants to terrorize.

The existing environment in Britain at that time also fed into this antipathy. That was a period when Enoch Powell's "Rivers of Blood" pronouncement was still fresh in the minds of at least a section of the British people. Enoch Powell was a Conservative Member of Parliament who, in a 1968 speech in Birmingham, had forewarned of extreme racial tension from unchecked immigration, opening up a Pandora's box of violent racism that viciously targeted immigrants:

> "*As I look ahead, I am filled with foreboding. Like the Roman, I seem to see "the River Tiber foaming with much blood". That tragic and intractable phenomenon which we watch with horror on the*

> *other side of the Atlantic but which there is interwoven with the history and existence of the States itself, is coming upon us here by our own volition and our own neglect. Indeed, it has all but come.In numerical terms, it will be of American proportions long before the end of the century. Only resolute and urgent action will avert it even now. Whether there will be the public will to demand and obtain that action, I do not know. All I know is that to see, and not to speak, would be the great betrayal.*"

Quoting statistics, Powell estimated that there would be 3.5 million immigrants in 15-20 years and the figure would touch 7 million by the turn of the century. His response to the situation was voluntary re-emigration:

> "*We must be mad, literally mad, as a nation to be permitting the annual inflow of some 50,000 dependants, who are for the most part the material of the future growth of the immigrant descended population. It is like watching a nation busily engaged in heaping up its own funeral pyre. So insane are we that we actually permit unmarried persons to immigrate for the purpose of founding a family with spouses and fiancées whom they have never seen.*"

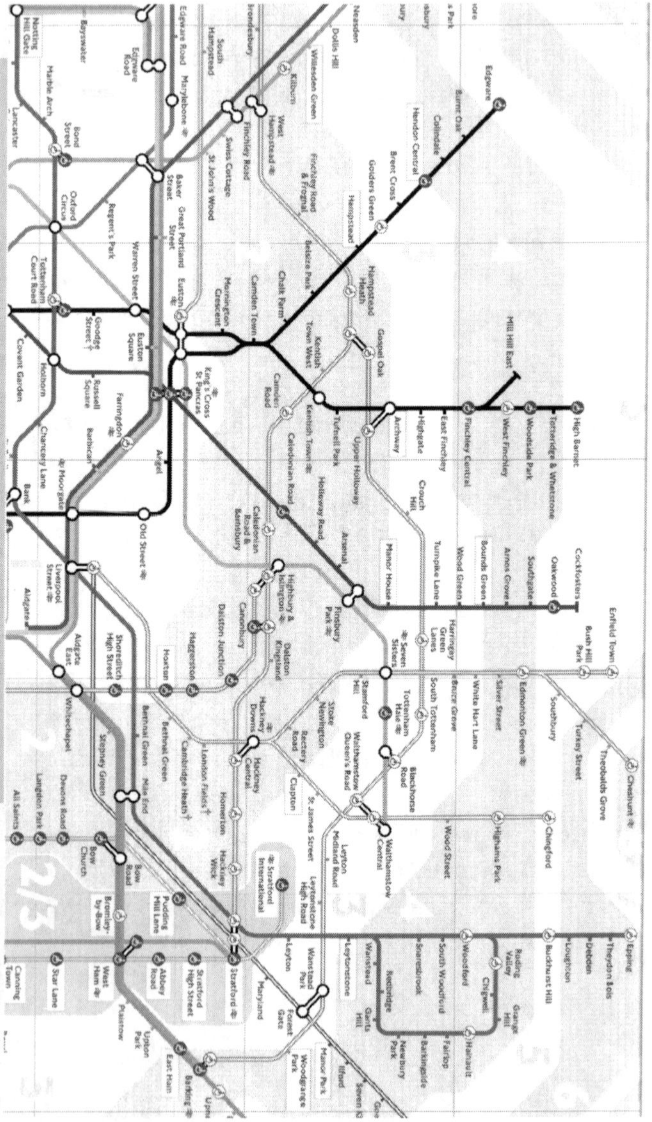

Fig 3:Truncated Map of London Underground

> *"I turn to re-emigration. If all immigration ended tomorrow, the rate of growth of the immigrant and immigrant-descended population would be substantially reduced, but the prospective size of this element in the population would still leave the basic character of the national danger unaffected. This can only be tackled while a considerable proportion of the total still comprises persons who entered this country during the last ten years or so. Hence the urgency of implementing now the second element of the Conservative Party's policy: the encouragement of re-emigration."*

Enoch Powell was promptly sacked from his position as Shadow Defence Secretary of the Conservative Party but the cat was out of the bag. There was a groundswell of public opinion in his favor, especially from the working class, and the stage was set for racism to flourish. In view of this growing popular support for Powell's viewpoint, a move to prosecute him officially was dropped.

Despite the punitive action by the Conservative Party leadership, there were certain quarters of the Conservative leadership that quietly sympathized with Powell's venomous outpouring. Among these tacit sympathizers, it was rumored, was Margaret Thatcher. And now Margaret Thatcher was at the helm of Great Britain, having been elected prime minister in 1979; the environment was certain to sour for immigrants especially from the subcontinent.

Adding fuel to the fire was an unenviable job market: in 1980, nearly 3 million Britons were unemployed; that is about 12.5 percent of the working population. Unemployment was mainly the result of economic recession and industry reorganization. But vested groups found a convenient scapegoat in immigrants.

Britain, despite a significant number of black and colored immigrants, was still an overwhelmingly white society. Whites constituted 92.1 percent of a total population of 56 million; Asians, a term that bracketed Indians, Pakistanis and Bangladeshis, made up barely 3.5 percent of the population.

Immigrants from India began arriving in the UK mainly after Indian independence in 1947. Prior to that there was negligible Indian presence in Great Britain. In 1939 there were no more than one hundred Indians in the entire city of Birmingham.

The first wave of Indian immigrants who landed in Britain in the 1950s did so to man blue-collar jobs that whites were unwilling to take up. These Indians found jobs as bus drivers and factory workers. Later, they moved on to establish the mom-and-pop corner shops that have now become a permanent fixture in the UK.

The second wave of significant immigration occurred between 1965 and 1972 when Idi Amin's brutal regime drove thousands of British passport holding Gujarati Indians to seek refuge in Great Britain. These Gujarati immigrants were descendants of laborers, clerks and low-level administrators who had been shipped to East Africa by the British Raj to carry out the menial tasks associated with the running of the Great British Empire.

The 1972 Immigration Act decreed that only holders of work permits or individuals with parents or grandparents born in the UK could enter the country, effectively curbing primary immigration. Physicians like me who were much-needed to fill the vacancies in the National Health Service fell under the purview of this Act.

Therefore Indian immigrants to the UK were not, by and large, uninvited guests who had snuck into the country illegally, but cheap labor encouraged by the authorities to meet their needs. Ironically, Enoch Powell, the high priest of anti-immigration was himself responsible for inviting doctors from Commonwealth countries to fill vacancies in the NHS when he was the health minister during the period 1960 to 1963. Therefore to turn on these immigrants in times of recession was a vile and repugnant act; a tendency, however, in keeping with the exploitative nature of the British people so clearly exemplified by colonialism.

I glanced at the raucous group through the corner of my eyes. They kept casting looks in my direction, gesticulating and making remarks. Initially I could not hear what they were saying but soon the remarks got louder, 'Paki' being the only discernible word that was repeated.

A welter of emotions gripped me as I tried to come to terms with this unexpected and unpleasant encounter in a new land. Looking back now, I realize how unprepared and reckless I had been when I had embarked on this venture to Great Britain. I had no idea of the social tensions that existed and shockingly had made no attempt to educate myself about this important facet of travel to a foreign land.

Initially I tried to ignore the skinheads pretending to be engrossed in my newspaper. But the chants only grew louder and louder, becoming more and more ugly. I looked around for any other passenger but there was none. The train meanwhile continued to rattle along rapidly through long dark tunnels, the jarring sound and external darkness only adding to my discomfiture. I desperately waited for the next stop hoping to get off, but the wait appeared endless. The train kept going on and on.

I felt like a prey being hunted. I moved towards the seat closest to the door ready to hop out at the next station. It was then that the group moved in on me. They got up from their seats and sauntered towards me mouthing profanities. They encircled me, the hefty looking one with the tattoo on his arm stood directly in front of me with the other two flanking him on either side. The girl stood a few feet away giggling incessantly stopping only to blow a bubble with the gum in her mouth. The boys taunted me, first softly and then more harshly, their tone full of rancor. Their garbled, accented speech prevented me from understanding exactly what they were saying. All that I could decipher was the word, "Paki" which they kept repeating. One of them spat in front of me qualifying his action with the words, "You dirty Paki." Another brought a menacing fist close to my face but didn't actually touch me.

Obviously, they were hoping to provoke me into a physical confrontation. I refused to take the bait. I don't know whether it was discretion or plain fright that kept me from responding to their jibes. I managed to keep my cool through it all. Luckily before the encounter became physically violent, the train lurched to a stop at a station. I dashed out through the door onto the platform outside, half expecting the skinheads to follow me. Fortunately they didn't and the train moved on leaving me standing on an empty platform, tremulous, frightened and alone.

I got into the next train, carefully choosing a crowded compartment. I was in a daze, badly shaken and traumatized. True, I had escaped a physical assault and was fortunate to be alive, unlike Dr Amal Dharry, a West Indian doctor of Asian origin who had been brutally stabbed to death in a fish and chips shop in Wolverhampton a few days earlier. But the effect on my psyche was profound and would persist throughout my two-and-a-half-years stay in Britain, infusing in me a sense of agoraphobia that was crippling at times.

Racial attacks continue to be the bane of Indian students traveling to Britain for higher studies. In the early hours of Boxing Day 2011, nearly 30 years after my own ugly experience, a young 23-year-old Indian student, Anuj Bidve was shot dead in Manchester in what appeared to be a pointless shooting. Anuj and his friends, who had inadvertently strayed into a crime-ridden area of Manchester, Ordsall, were accosted by two young white men who put a gun to Anuj's head and pulled the trigger for no apparent reason.

Anuj had arrived in Britain only three months earlier and had been studying microelectronics at Lancaster University. His family back in Pune (earlier Poona), India, was devastated. They just could not make any sense of this killing. This murder is another reminder that racism is never far from the surface of life in Britain. This incident also brings to the fore the profound ignorance among Indians of the reality of Britain: they continue to harbor glowing unrealistic pictures of civility and discipline carried over from colonial times in their minds.

Another incident reported in the media indicates how little things have changed in the last 30 years since I left the country. Racism against Indians is a fact of daily life in Britain today as the following news report from 2012 suggests. Strangely enough, the racial incident highlighted by the report occurred on the London Underground almost exactly at the same place where I was subject to an ugly race rant in 1980.

> "*A London Underground passenger has been jailed for 21 weeks after she admitted hurling racist abuse at fellow passengers. Jacqueline Woodhouse, 42, of Romford, east London, directed an expletive-ridden rant at Tube passengers on the Central line on 23 January (2011).*
>
> *A seven-minute video of the verbal assault was uploaded to YouTube.*
>
> *The video shows Galbant Juttla, who filmed the incident on his mobile phone, telling Woodhouse to keep her mouth shut and that she had had too much to drink.*
>
> *"It's not your country anyway so what's your problem?" she said.*
>
> *"It's been overtaken by people like you."*
>
> *In further remarks, on a packed train between St Paul's and Mile End stations, she told passengers: "I'll have you arrested because you don't live here" and "I hope you are not claiming benefits*"

(*BBC News* website).

The effect of my unpleasant encounter on the Tube train restricted my outdoor adventures considerably. I began spending more and more time within the precincts of the hospital.

The duration of my locum in Epping was six weeks. Three weeks into my job I was already scouting for the next one, immersing myself in a ritual that I would be repeating innumerable times over the next two years: waiting eagerly for the *BMJ* every week, scouring the last few pages for suitable jobs, locum or permanent, sending out copies of my résumé and waiting expectantly for a positive response. It was a nerve-racking experience, with the level of tension mounting with each passing day as the end date approached.

What would I do if I didn't get a job? Where would I go? Where would I stay? These were the questions that kept swirling in my head during those days. I didn't have an independent place to stay. Jobs came with living accommodation. If I had no job, it meant no place to stay as well.

With a week left to go in my job at Epping, I landed a position at East Birmingham Hospital. It was for a period of 10 days and at the level of a house officer, one step lower than my present rank. Nevertheless, I was overjoyed, for it was in a specialty that I wanted: internal medicine. Dr Roy, my consultant in Epping, tried to induce me to stay at Epping by offering me a permanent position as a senior house officer, but I demurred. I had no intention of getting stuck in a dead-end career in geriatrics. It was a decision that many of my friends and acquaintances dubbed as foolhardy. Who would pass up a regular position for a 10-day locum? The logic appeared ridiculous. But I was not willing to compromise. Six weeks later, I left Epping and headed for Birmingham with the hope that my gamble would payoff...

CHAPTER SEVEN

A Harrowing Weekend On-Call and an Awkward Introduction

It then dawned on me. I was the doctor on call for the weekend. Stupid of me not to realize that. After all what are locums hired for?

He broke off his sentence mid-stream, turned to me with a benevolent smile and asked politely, "Where are you from, sir?"

"Epping," I blurted out without realizing the incongruity of such a response coming as it were from a brown-skinned house officer.

He paused for a moment, the irritation clearly showing on his face, and then persisted, "I mean originally."

The fare was an attractive 2 pounds one-way. That cinched my decision. I opted for a bus ride to Birmingham rather than a rail journey, overriding my preference for the latter. Being strapped to a bus seat for a maximum of three hours was not going to be that unbearable, I convinced myself. Birmingham is located about 100 miles to the northwest of London, and the bus driver assured me that we would be there in two and a half hours barring any traffic jams.

Birmingham at first sight was quite different, much quieter and lacked the bustling energy and variety of London. Not to say that it was not culturally diverse. It had one of the largest concentrations of Asians in Britain: Asians formed nearly a fifth of its total population. It was also UK's second-largest city and was once a center of great importance being the hub of the Industrial Revolution in the eighteenth century. Nevertheless it now lacked the verve noticeable in London.

East Birmingham Hospital was a large district general hospital located in the eastern part of the city as the name implied, and was much bigger than the provincial hospital in Epping. Today, it has been rechristened as Heartlands Hospital. The hospital complex itself consisted of several independent pre-War buildings spread out over a few acres of land. Though the distance between the various buildings was not great, it did pose a problem during snow-ridden days.

When I arrived there late in the evening I was informed that the doctors' quarters were all taken and I was to be accommodated in the nurses' hostel. To say that my lodging was modest is an overstatement. It was literally a closet, a

6 feet by 8 feet room that had no windows or ventilation of any sort. The only source of light was a 40-Watt bulb high up in the ceiling. A small twin-sized bed filed the entirety of the room, leaving little space to move around. You either went straight to bed or got out of the room. Its location at the end of a dark, dingy corridor added to its cheerless character.

But I was in no mood to complain. Hailing from a poverty-stricken Third World country that India then was, I just lacked the gumption to protest. Moreover I was excited at the prospect of beginning a job in the specialty that I wanted. I was not going to mar my prospects by grumbling about relatively trivial matters. I consoled myself with the thought that I was going to be there for only 10 days.

With regard to my actual job, I hit the ground running. By the time I reached the hospital it was late Friday afternoon and most of the workforce had already left for the weekend. The outgoing physician handed me a battered pager taped together with cellophane and disappeared promptly. It then dawned on me. I was the doctor on call for the weekend. Stupid of me not to realize that. After all what are locums hired for?

To begin a new job in a new place is a daunting proposition. But to be on call as your very first assignment is enough to take anyone's breath away. I faced the situation not like a warrior going to battle but like a helpless lamb being taken to slaughter. And slaughtered I was that weekend.

It was a horrendous nightmare. The pager never ceased to beep, going off incessantly from 5 p.m. on Friday evening to 9 a.m. on Monday morning, a marathon stretch of 64 hours. No sooner had I answered one call and was about to rest than the beeper went off again demanding my immediate attention. The tally of the calls that I received during those two days was close to 200.

Compared to modern pagers which come equipped with a display screen that flashes a message complete with the telephone number of the caller, devices in those days were ancient, with no such capability. All that the pager did was to make a monotonous and irritating beeping sound over and over again. One could not even modulate the ringtone or switch to a vibrate mode to escape the irksome sound.

The limited capability of those pagers made the task of answering a page a two-step process. First you called the operator to find out who was looking for you and then you called the ward that needed you. Sometimes you were left hanging for minutes together with no response from the other end, adding to your frustration and anger.

"If the floor wants my services so badly at 2 a.m., they had better answer me when I call," I grumbled to myself countless times during that two-day period.

To add to that, all the medical wards were not in one location as I mentioned earlier, but spread out in different buildings that were a fair distance apart with no connecting conduit. Getting to these sites meant walking in the open, bracing the wintry cold and darkness of the night. With no idea of the topography of the hospital, I was completely at sea, losing my direction repeatedly. Several times at night I landed up in the wrong ward only to be told that the place I was required to be was at the other end forcing me to trek all the way back. This can be really frustrating when it happens at 2.30 a.m.

As a house officer you belong to the bottom of the totem pole and are required to perform all menial tasks without so much as a murmur of protest. No sympathy is expected and no sympathy is given. It is a rite of passage that newly-trained physicians have to undergo. Period.

Most of my work that weekend involved routine tasks like rewriting orders or inserting intravenous lines, mundane from a young physician's perspective but an important part of the training process. There were no computerized medical records then that enabled you to belt out orders simultaneously to four different wards from the comfort of your room. Every single order required your physical presence in the ward and your legible autograph. An hour's work from that era can be condensed into a few minutes of work today with little scope for error, as the automated system promptly corrects your mistakes.

The task of writing an order appears simple, a one-line communiqué that tells the nurse what to do or what medicine to administer. But each element of this directive is open to error. The name of the drug has to be written legibly, the dose has to be correct, and the manner of administration such as oral, intravenous, subcutaneous, intramuscular or rectal, has to be right. A slip-up in any one of these components can spell disaster for the patient and the physician.

This excerpt from a *Time* magazine report in 2007 ("Cause of Death: Sloppy Doctors" by Jeremy Caplan) outlines the significance of this problem.

> "*Doctors' sloppy handwriting kills more than 7,000 people annually. It's a shocking statistic, and, according to a July 2006 report from the National Academies of Science's Institute of Medicine (IOM), preventable medication mistakes also injure more than 1.5 million Americans annually. Many*

> *such errors result from unclear abbreviations and dosage indications and illegible writing on some of the 3.2 billion prescriptions written in the U.S. every year.*
>
> *To address the problem — and give the push for electronic medical records a shove - a coalition of health-care companies and technology firms will launch a program Tuesday to enable all doctors in the US to write electronic prescriptions for free. The National e-prescribing Patient Safety Initiative (NEPSI) will offer doctors access to eRxNow, a Web-based tool that physicians can use to write prescriptions electronically, check for potentially harmful drug interactions and, ensure that pharmacies provide appropriate medications and dosages.*"

But in those days we had no such statistics. Our ideas of the extent of such errors were based on anecdotes exchanged over the dinner table or in informal conversations. A colleague informed you in a hushed tone of how a fellow house officer nearly killed a patient by a rapid push of intravenous potassium as opposed to a slow infusion, while another recalled in what would seem as cruel humor to a layman the travails of a patient who had been wrongly administered Lasix (a diuretic that increases your urinary frequency) instead of Losec (an anti-ulcer medication), the error emanating from the illegible scrawl of a sleepy house officer's pen.

Any formal assessment of "Quality"was alien to the field of medicine then. There were no forums to discuss physician errors, no tools to measure them and no plans to reduce mistakes. The closest we had to a quality control monitor was the stern head nurse who watched over you like a hawk, especially if you happened to be a house officer. There was no dearth of such head nurses in East Birmingham and was I happy about that.

By Saturday evening, after nearly 24 hours continuously on the job, I had reached a point of mental and physical exhaustion. I had managed to get barely an hour of sleep. I had become a zombie, a mechanical robot with little capacity left for discriminative thought. But for the watchful eyes of the head nurse, I am sure I would have committed several blunders.

The head nurse of a ward was both a bane and boon. Yes, she kept a watchful eye over young house officers like me preventing us from making embarrassing mistakes. But the protection came at a cost. Every "t" had to be crossed and every "i" to be dotted before one could get a moment of respite. The slightest lapse resulted in one trekking back to the ward to rectify the mistake.

Every call is an experience in itself taking you through a cycle of emotions, the degree of each emotion experienced depending on one's stress level. Early enthusiasm and excitement is soon replaced by a matter-of-fact business approach. As the energy level ebbs, equanimity can no longer be maintained and irritability sets in, punctuated by spasms of suppressed rage triggered by seemingly harmless events. But don't get me wrong. These are internal convolutions that are very rarely discernible on the outside and seldom affect a physician's professional performance. The penultimate emotion is one of apathetic resignation. As Monday morning approaches, hope stirs some life into you and finally relief, that orgasmic moment when you hand over the dreaded pager to the next physician on call.

Boy, was I relieved when I handed over the beeper to my transient colleague that Monday morning!

He was tall, easily over 6 feet, distinguished looking and some would say even handsome for his age. Clad in a gray suit under a physician's white coat he was busy demonstrating the cruel effects of rheumatoid arthritis on the proximal interphalangeal joint (the joint closest to the base of your finger) when I stumbled in to join the rounds, already a few minutes late and still dazed from the weekend call.

He broke off his sentence in mid-stream, turned to me with a benevolent smile and asked politely, "Where are you from, sir?"

"Epping," I blurted out without realizing the incongruity of such a response coming as it were from a brown-skinned Indian or Asian house officer.

He froze paused for a moment, the irritation clearly showing on his face, and then persisted., "I mean originally," ." he persisted.

"From India." I said.

It was the 1980s, the world was still relatively insular and I suppose the English consultant could be excused for his pattern of questioning which was obviously prompted by the color of my skin. However 30 years later despite a vastly changed global environment, diehard British attitudes like this appear not to have changed. Even if you have been born and brought up in Britain and know no other land other than Britain and no other language other than English, you are still subject to uncomfortable questioning because of your color, as this excerpt from an article titled, "Tired of being asked where I am from" by Ariane Sherine which appeared in *The Guardian*in March 2010 (nearly 30 years after my experiences in the UK) indicates.

> "*So here's a ready-made answer for the overly curious. Last weekend, I had The Conversation for the 3,897th time — and this time, it took place in central London just two roads away from the hospital where I was born. As usual, it went like this:*
>
> *Stranger: Where are you from? (Translation: You look a bit brown. Why are you brown?)*
>
> *Me: London.*
>
> *Stranger: No, where are you really from? (Translation: You are clearly telling me untruths. Brown people do not come from London.)*
>
> *Me: London.*
>
> *Stranger (exasperated): No, where are your parents from? (Translation: Now you're just being obtuse.)*
>
> *Me: Africa and America.*
>
> *Stranger (confused): Erm...so where are your family from, like, back in the day? (Translation: People who come from Africa and America do not look like you.)*
>
> *Me: Iran, India, Africa, America and England.*
>
> *Stranger (relieved): India and Iran! Do you ever go back?*
>
> *At this point, I have to explain that it's hard to go back to somewhere you have never been. I've lived in London since I was a zygote, have a London*

accent and don't speak any languages except English — yet just because I'm cashew-coloured, I'm often questioned about my heritage."

Despite this awkward introduction, my subsequent interaction with Dr Howard-Williams, that was the consultant's name, was without incident. Dr Howard-Williams was a kindly gentleman who spoke in a soft polite tone that exuded genuine empathy. He had a special interest in rheumatology or joint diseases. Accordingly, his ward consisted of mostly patients with joint diseases. The burden of arthritis in the UK is enormous and imposes a hefty strain on society. Arthritis is in fact the most common cause among people receiving Disability Living Allowance (DLA) in the UK. No wonder rheumatology, unlike in India was an important subject and a distinct specialty.

My exposure to joint diseases during my training in India was limited. Arthritis in India was not a common medical student topic as in the UK and the chronic nature of the diseases made it an item of less priority; infectious diseases and other life-threatening disorders took precedence. Rheumatology was a little bit of a novelty for me and I found the rounds fairly interesting. I would be less than honest if I used any other term stronger than that to describe my feelings for this field. Rheumatology by nature was pedestrian, not glamorous like cardiology or cardiac surgery and even less exciting than specialties that concentrated on the digestive system or lung problems.

Nevertheless, Dr Howard-Williams was a good teacher and I learnt a lot from him in those two weeks that I spent on his unit. Specifically, I learnt how to differentiate between rheumatoid arthritis and osteoarthritis, the two main commonly encountered joint problems.

Dr Williams was the epitome of English punctuality. He started rounds exactly at 9 a.m. and was very particular that every member of his team be there on time. The team itself consisted of three other physicians apart from me. There was Tom Waitman, the senior registrar who appeared perpetually tired and had good reason to be. He was nearly 40 years old, with thining hair, and was yet to land a consultant position. All his energy was consumed in looking for one. He was the friendliest of the lot and one who came across as truly good at heart.

Nice is not a word that I would use to describe the other two: civil, but definitely not nice. Next in the hierarchy was John Smith, the registrar, a red-haired Englishman with a goatee who was extremely uptight on rounds but who did loosen up once Dr Williams had left the scene. He had been to India once and made it a point to comment on the inefficiency and corruptness of the Indian bureaucracy whenever he got a chance. The last member of the team was Mindy Turcot the SHO who constantly peered at me through large thick glasses, was physically on the heavy side and did not stand out as being particularly knowledgeable with regard to medicine.

Rounds usually lasted for about three hours but on some days could go on for four to five hours with a break for lunch between two sessions. Rounds were not confined to medical topics and frequently the conversation veered to include local issues and international politics. Without such distractions, rounds can become unbearable especially towards the fag end.

Dr Williams, like many English consultants, was a frequent visitor in a professional capacity to many of Britain's former colonies. Libya's Muammar Al-Gaddafi was at the height of his eccentricity in the 80s and Dr Williams had just returned from a trip to Libya. He spent a good half hour one day recalling his recent visit there, regaling us with details of camel jaunts into the desert and telling us of how he had made his displeasure explicitly known to his local contacts with regard to Gaddafi's wayward ways, in particular his repressive policies.

Post-rounds banter was also interesting, sometimes even more interesting than the rounds themselves. Juicy tidbits surfaced that could not be voiced on rounds. It was a free-for-all. No topic or individual was off limits. A gossip piece doing the rounds was that Dr Williams had just married someone 20 years his junior and was desperately trying to keep in shape to match her age. Whether this was true or not I never really was able to confirm. Sexual peccadilloes of junior doctors and nurses were another staple item with specific events often being described in great detail and with relish.

Life beyond the hospital was lazy and slow-paced. With no car to move around and still chary of venturing out alone after my London encounter with skinheads, I spent a great deal of my time in the library studying for my exam or in the doctors' lounge watching TV.

The doctors' lounge in a British hospital is a hub where junior doctors congregate after work hours. It forms a convenient meeting spot for single young doctors especially locum physicians like myself who have no family or permanent quarters to go back to after work. It is a place that infuses a sense of camaraderie among locum physicians.

A locum is a lonely figure. Loneliness, even when temporary, makes one vulnerable; there is a pressing urge to foster new relationships. But there is a glitch: relationships formed during locum tenures are fleeting, ending as abruptly as they begin. Surprisingly, in the 10 days that I spent in Birmingham I got to know several physicians quite well. Each one had an interesting story to tell, where they were in their life's journey and where they intended to go.

There were a good number of Indian physicians among the locum community at East Birmingham Hospital during my stay there. One of the physicians was Jeevan Mehta, an affable young man who hailed from Gujarat. Bubbly and humorous, he embodied the phrase joie de vivre. However he had one regret: he had whiled away his time in the UK so far "chasing student nurses" as he put it, instead of studying. Now he wanted to pass his exam, the dreaded FRCS, the main purpose of his coming to the UK. He had seen me frequenting the library and felt that associating with me would somehow make him more studious and less vulnerable to temptation, thereby helping him achieve his goal.

Then there was Rita Kumar who was doing a locum in orthopedics, a rather unusual career choice for a female physician at that time. Her husband too was a physician; he worked in Walsall, a mid-sized town located a few miles to the north of Birmingham.

Rita was tall and graceful, strikingly pretty with chiseled features; her smile was radiant and disarming. She was well informed, intelligent and an engaging conversationalist; it was a pleasure talking to her at the breakfast table where I often bumped into her more by design than chance. Later, I learnt that she had returned to India to provide much-needed medical care to village folk living in remote areas, churned out a few novels that had rural India as the backdrop and came to be well known for both her writing and praiseworthy medical mission.

Jaymanne was a microbiologist from Sri Lanka who was working on a PhD thesis. He was a pensive individual but quite friendly when one got to know him better. We had many a conversation on a wide range of topics that included politics and radical social movements. Although I never explicitly asked the question and he never said so in unequivocal terms, I gathered that he was one of those young men who were smitten by the extreme leftist movement that was a rage across the subcontinent in those times.

The 70s and 80s was a period that saw hordes of brilliant young men and women in the subcontinent give up their studies to join armed struggles that drew inspiration from the Russian and Chinese model, only to be disillusioned later. I had a classmate in medical school, an absolutely brilliant student from a privileged background, who had abandoned his studies in Delhi to join this "noble cause". Rumor had it that his influential father had then pressed into service a veritable posse and spent a fortune to rescue his son from the clutches of the Naxalites (a leftist radical group in India). Subsequently, this classmate of mine had been banished to medical school in South India far away from the influence of these extremists.

I had a faint suspicion that Jaymanne too had ideas of joining such a movement on his return to Sri Lanka. But for the present he seemed to be living a placid lifestyle complete with a comfortable live-in arrangement, his companion being a pretty young nurse of Indian origin from the Caribbean. They were kind enough to invite me for an enjoyable dinner one night, taking special care to cook vegetarian dishes bearing my preference in mind. Compared to the drab cafeteria food, any other type of food was welcome; I found the coconut-based curries that are the specialty of Sri Lankan cuisine especially appetizing.

It was early November as I neared the end of my 10-day stint in East Birmingham Hospital. The days were getting shorter, darkness was setting in earlier and there was a nip in the air. By the time I got off from work around 4 p.m., it was pitch dark. It was difficult to step outside without a padded jacket or some piece of warm clothing. Hailing from the southern part of India where normal temperatures routinely hover around 100 degrees Fahrenheit, and thus, unused to heavy attire, I found this requirement uncomfortable and restrictive, but I had little choice. The few times that I did venture out without an overcoat, I found myself shivering uncontrollably; my teeth broke into a chatter, my lips became heavy, and exhaled air formed a visible plume whenever I tried to say something, forcing me to withdraw into the warmth of the indoors. In short, the picture outside was depressing: gray, gloomy, cold and uninviting.

On the job front I had managed to arrange another locum at East Birmingham Hospital as an SHO in hematology for a period of one week. Locums were much easier to obtain through direct personal interaction as opposed to applications through mail or telephonic contact. I had landed this locum by directly approaching the concerned consultant one afternoon when he happened to be making rounds in the same ward that I was posted in. Dr Connolly, the hematology consultant, who was much shorter than Dr Williams but more agile, sized me up from head to foot for a moment, asked me how long I had worked with Dr Williams, and told me that the job was mine even before I could respond to his query.

But that position did not start till late November. Between the end of my present locum and that one, there was a hiatus of two long weeks. With barely a day to go, relief came my way. My uncle's friend who went by the initials ASK had cajoled a colleague of his to offer me an SHO locum that would bridge this gap. Hastily I stuffed my meager belongings into that rickety old suitcase that I had brought from India, the only constant companion of my itinerant status and headed for the next stop: Mansfield, Nottinghamshire.

My posting in Mansfield was a lackluster one with no memorable incidents. The geriatric ward that I worked in was a long-stay unit for the elderly that was not meant to handle even the mildest of emergencies. Hospitals like this one were not real hospitals in the true sense of the word. They acted as "relief centers" that provided temporary respite for families from the onerous task of caring for the old, especially when they had to go out of town or on a vacation. Accordingly, the inmates here had few issues that demanded immediate attention. Moreover, at the slightest hint of medical instability, patients were promptly shipped out to the local general hospital.

I was left with little to do. Every morning I religiously made my rounds, mechanically repeating the same orders day after day and waiting patiently for my consultant Dr Hassan to make rounds with me. Dr Hassan was a portly balding man in his 60s and had been trained in Bangladesh. But that was for him a distant memory, having lived in the UK for over 30 years. He was kind to me and treated me with great respect and I was deeply grateful to him for this locum. While this job did not provide me with any professional satisfaction, it gave me something to do, netted me a few pounds and, more importantly, provided me with a roof over my head.

On my last day in Mansfield, a major snowstorm hit the region. It was my first experience of snow and I was both excited and curious. All morning it was dark and cloudy; the sun was nowhere to be seen. Temperatures plummeted to sub-zero levels and people stayed indoors for the most part. The actual snowfall started around 2 PM in the afternoon: it began with light rain interspersed with sleet which then turned into snow. Initially the flakes were small- tiny white flecks with a feathery appearance that danced in the air capriciously according to the vagaries of the wind; some hanging motionlessly for a brief moment before floating gracefully to the ground beneath. Watching this snow for the first time in my life from the warm comfort of my uncle's friend ASK's living room, I was entranced. I had moved into his house in preparation for the snowstorm.

At first the snow did not stick; the flakes melted instantaneously as they hit the ground leaving no trace behind. A faint dusting collected on tree branches and the roofs, giving them a freshly-washed appearance. By 3 PM, the intensity of the snowfall increased. Flakes no longer dissolved on touching the ground, they accumulated, covering everything in sight with a blanket of white – a mesmerizing sight for someone who has never seen snow before.

I bundled myself into a warm jacket, covered my face with a muffler, put on leather gloves and ventured out into the open. I wanted to touch the snow, hold it in my hands to see how it felt. I picked up a small handful and attempted to roll it into a ball, but it melted as soon as I closed my fist. I waited for some time for the snow to get heavier and picked up a larger lump of snow. This time it did not melt - a small snowball formed in my glove. Excited, I threw it into the air like a little child. All around me, I saw children frolicking in the snow, targeting each other with snowballs, coasting down inclines on snow sleds

As evening approached the snowfall progressed, coming down faster and heavier. Visibility dimmed to less than 30 feet with a sheet of white opacity obscuring my vision. Everyone moved indoors. An eerie silence enveloped the scene outside, occasionally disturbed by the creaking sound of tree branches falling to the ground under the weight of wet snow. Throughout the evening and night, the snowfall continued until everything in sight was covered with a blanket of white snow - sidewalks, roads, roof tops, cars parked on streets. Evergreen trees covered with snow resembled the pictures I had seen in children's books.

All night, I could hear the mechanical drone of snow plough machines as they went about their job of clearing the snow from the roads. Local residents dutifully cleaned their respective sidewalks as best as they could, creating an ambulatory path from the debris of snow flanked on each side by a wall of displaced snow at least two feet in height. Their promptness and sincerity was admirable.

As I watched the snow piling up outside, my anxiety mounted. How was I going to reach Birmingham by 8 AM the next morning? I was supposed to report for duty at East

Birmingham Hospital the following day. With no personal mode of transport and bus services temporarily suspended, I was in a quandary. To add to my misfortune, Mansfield did not have its own rail station; the closest station that would connect me to Birmingham was Nottingham, a good 30 miles away.

Luckily, ASK came to my rescue. Not only was he the perfect host that evening, but he also drove me to the rail station at 2 a.m. in the morning despite the raging snowstorm. I will always treasure the generosity of people like ASK who went out of their way to help me, especially when I was passing through a trying time. The help that one receives when one is down and out is what one values the most

CHAPTER EIGHT

THIRD WORLD LONDON

With a flourish, he whipped out a chest X-ray from the cart that the head nurse was pushing along as we made rounds, held it up against the light of the window and turned to me as though seeking my opinion – which in reality was a test of my proficiency. The clear lucidness of the lung had been replaced by smudges of opacity signifying fibrotic damage. "TB," I blurted out.

If one is dropped onto the grimy garbage strewn streets of Hackney from the skies above, one cannot believe that this is a part of London or England. Hackney, located in north London, qualifies as one of the most deprived inner city areas of UK. Unemployment traditionally runs high. Hackney was especially hard hit by the global financial crisis in 2008, forcing nearly one in five of its residents to seek a government dole. More than 50 percent of its citizenry lives in socially rented accommodation compared, to 19.2 percent nationwide. Crime rates are scary. In nearly every category, be it minor theft, burglary or an automobile related offence, Hackney surpasses the national average.

Even back in 1981, it was not a desirable place to venture into. However at that time I was blissfully ignorant of the harsh reality of Hackney. Furthermore I really had no choice. I gratefully accepted whatever locum that came my way. And to be honest, I was quite excited at the prospect of doing a three-week locum in general medicine at Hackney Hospital because of its affiliation with the prestigious St Bartholomew's Hospital or "Barts" as it is commonly referred to within the medical fraternity.

Although St Bartholomew's Hospital has fallen on bad days in recent times (there was talk of closure in the 1990s), it has, through the ages, been revered as a fine institution of medical learning with a history dating back to 1123 when it was founded as a sanctuary for the ill. The likes of William Harvey, the discoverer of blood circulation, and Elizabeth Blackwell, the first woman physician in the UK, graced its portals enhancing its reputation. For a young physician with an academic bent of mind like me, the idea of working even on the periphery of such an illustrious institution was exciting enough.

Compared to St Bartholomew's, Hackney Hospital was more recent in its origin, having started as a one-room infirmary for the poor in 1750. Although it expanded over the years to become a larger hospital, it carried a stigma and ordinary people were loath to seek care at this hospital. As in the past, it continued to cater to the lowest economic strata of the locality, which had changed over the years to include blacks and immigrants who now constituted its main patient base.

With blacks and immigrants forming a significant portion of the patient population, it was natural to encounter diseases that one saw in Third World countries. No wonder that the first case we discussed on my first day in Hackney Hospital was a man with tuberculosis. The patient, I recall, was an elderly black gentleman, gaunt beyond imagination; the contours of his bony skeleton were clearly visible beneath his stretched ebony skin. He had appeared at the outpatient clinic a day earlier complaining of having lost 20 pounds over a 2-month period. He had been promptly admitted to the hospital for further investigation.

Dr Newton, my consultant for the next three weeks, was a dedicated senior physician who had spent his entire career at Hackney Hospital. He belonged to the old school that reveled in bedside clinical medicine as opposed to the technology-based investigational emphasis that is in vogue today. With a flourish, he whipped out a chest X-ray from the cart that the head nurse was pushing along as we made rounds, held it up against the light of the window and turned to me as though seeking my opinion – which in reality was a test of my proficiency. The clear lucidness of the lung had been replaced by smudges of opacity signifying fibrotic damage. “TB,” I blurted out without a second thought using the well- known abbreviation for tuberculosis. Dr Newton was visibly impressed. First impressions, like anywhere else, do matter in the medical field as well. I sailed through the three weeks of my locum appointment without any problems.

My sojourn at the hospital was notable for interaction with physicians from other parts of the world. So far I had come across physicians from the subcontinent and local

English physicians. Here at Hackney I met physicians from other countries such as Nigeria and Sudan and my contact with them added to my knowledge of these countries.

Tom Barki was a Christian from Nigeria and it was through him that I first came to know that Nigeria is almost equally divided into an Islamic north and Christian south. Nigeria had been a British colony till 1960 when it was granted independence, and had a large body of educated professionals as a result of the English system of schooling that had been introduced during the British period. Tom obviously was a product of such schooling as he spoke perfect English.

Tom was a registrar and my immediate boss. Soft-spoken and polite, he was more of an introvert and I rarely saw him in the doctors' lounge which serves as a watering hole for physicians after hours. Making rounds with Tom at work was a breeze as he was not the fault-finding type who are on a constant watch for the minutest of lapses. He was more of the "teaching type," given to medical homilies that tended to be a little lengthy at times and sometimes even mildly annoying, especially around lunchtime when your stomach takes over your mind.

Like me, he had his eyes set on America; he had cleared his required exams and was waiting for his paperwork to come through.

My first encounter with a physician from Sudan was not a pleasant one. It occurred one evening as I strolled into the doctors' lounge to while away those long lonely evening hours. Trying to be congenial, I introduced myself as being from India to a group of physicians who were chatting with each other over a mug of beer, only to be met with an abrupt and rude retort from one of them. He was tall, with an Afro-cut and a wheat-brown complexion.

I would learn later that he hailed from Sudan. Without even acknowledging my greeting, he abrasively remarked: “India? Isn’t that the place they kill Muslims?”

He was obviously referring to the notorious Hindu-Muslim riots that occur frequently in India. Although taken aback, my first reaction was to launch into a spirited defense of my country enlightening the worthy of the fact that India happened to harbor one of the largest Muslim populations in the world and to explain to him the dynamics of Hindu-Muslim altercations. But on second thoughts, I decided against it. After a hard day’s work I was in no mood to engage in rancorous banter. I decided to ignore his provocative remark and moved on to settle down with a newspaper. From then on, I made it a point to avoid this physician.

My living accommodation for the two-week period was a hole in the wall, 8 feet by 6 feet in size and along a windowless corridor, very similar to the room that I had at the East Birmingham Hospital. I had to pinch myself several times to remind myself that I was in London and not Birmingham. Fortunately, this accommodation was located within the premises of the hospital and saved me from venturing out onto the unfriendly streets of Hackney, something that I was not eager to do. I don’t recall having stepped out of the hospital even once during the entire three-week tenure of my locum there.

This self-imposed confinement made my evenings long and dreary, providing me with ample time to subject myself to harsh self-recrimination for the uncertain state of my career and indulge in oodles of self-pity. It was on one of those evenings as I was walking down one of the gloomy corridors of the hospital on my way back to my room that I bumped into Cherian.

Cherian was carrying two paper cartons with signature wire handles that indicated their Chinese takeout origin. In true Indian tradition, after a brief introduction, he invited me to share his dinner. Over the next few days we got to know each other better.

Cherian was in his late 40s, much older than me, and had been a senior faculty member in cardiology at a prestigious Christian institution in south India for 15 years. His previous job, while professionally satisfying, paid poorly. The amount that he earned was just not sufficient to provide a decent living for his wife and two teenage sons. So he had decided to leave the country to seek greener pastures abroad and had landed up in Hackney Hospital where he now worked as a registrar in geriatrics.

This transition was clearly a step down in his professional career. But with regards to income it was a big leap forward. Even a registrar (a relatively low-ranking position that requires barely two years of post-medical school experience) in the UK was paid much better than a senior faculty with 15 years of experience at an Indian medical school. A registrar's annual salary in 1980 was a modest £15,000 which at the then prevailing exchange rate translated into 300,000 Indian rupees: a princely sum that would take Cherian five years to earn back home.

Being young, immature and unmarried, I could not bring myself to appreciate or understand this sort of a compromise. For me, a switch from a highly desirable specialty like cardiology to something banal like geriatrics was incomprehensible. In a perverse way, comparing his situation to mine made me feel a little better. At least I was still in my late 20s and had my entire career ahead of me, unlike Cherian who was pushing 50 years and still uncertain of where his career or life was headed. It made me realize the value of looking at life in relative terms.

But Cherian's plight also filled me with a sense of foreboding. What if I was destined to become the next Cherian, still searching for my calling at the age of 50? What if I never got a spot in the specialty that I liked - internal medicine? What if I never made it to the US? What if I became another statistic working in the isolated geriatric hospitals of Britain that were the dumping grounds for hordes of unsuccessful foreign physicians who were unable to make it into the specialties of their choice? Could I escape from the inequity of the British National Health Service to a more fair system across the pond?

Questions like these constantly reverberated through my mind, especially at times when even the immediate future seemed uncertain. With barely a week left for my job in Hackney to end, I still had no new job to go to and I was getting desperate.

Hackney was my sixth locum position in as many months. The year was coming to an end. It was Christmas time outside with all the glitzy decorations and merriment but I sat in my drab windowless room filling out the last of those 50 or so applications that had to be mailed out by the next working day. Maybe one of them would get me to where I wanted to go. Maybe...

CHAPTER NINE

The 'Iron Lady's' Vision of UK No Place for Asians

But all his pleading for Asians to be included in Margaret Thatcher's vision of a future UK came to naught; they hit a stone wall. The "Iron Lady" did not wilt or exhibit any compassion.

The anchor's crestfallen face at the end of the interview embodied the plight of the South Asian in Britain then: permanent rejection from British society after having spent a lifetime in that country.

The TV became my faithful companion during lonely evening hours and long listless weekends. It was inevitable that with such a high dose of exposure to news and current events that I would become an avid follower of local political happenings. Politically, Britain in 1980 was passing through an exciting phase, albeit a trifle rocky.

A year earlier in 1979, Margaret Thatcher had been elected as the first woman prime minister of Britain. She had led her party to a decisive victory over Labour headed by the previous Prime Minister James Callaghan. The 1979 election would prove to be a watershed in British politics for yet another reason: it was the beginning of 18 years of uninterrupted Conservative rule.

As a person, Margaret Thatcher was not an immensely popular figure. In fact in the polls leading up to the election, voters had indicated a preference for James Callaghan, the incumbent prime minister, despite an overall Conservative lead. In the end, however, Labour's poor governing record that had triggered a succession of strikes in 1978–79 – commonly referred to as the "winter of discontent" – sealed James Callaghan's fate and catapulted Margaret Thatcher to the top post.

Somewhere along her political career Margaret Thatcher had acquired the reputation of being a tough no-nonsense politician. A particularly strident indictment of the Soviet Union when she was the leader of the Opposition had resulted in a strong rebuke in the Soviet Defence Ministry newspaper which had dubbed her "The Iron Lady".

It was an epithet that would stick and one that Margaret Thatcher gladly exploited to her advantage. In the December of 1979 in a foreign policy speech delivered in New York Margaret Thatcher had affirmed her strong opposition to the policies of the Soviet Union and had willingly accepted the tag affixed to her:

> "*The immediate threat from the Soviet Union is military rather than ideological. The threat is not only to our security in Europe and North America but also, both directly and by proxy, in the third world. I have often spoken about the military challenge which the West faces today. I have sometimes been deliberately misunderstood, especially by my enemies who have labeled me the "Iron Lady." They are quite right - I am.*"

She went on to say:

> "*We can argue about Soviet motives. But the fact is that the Russians have the weapons and are getting more of them. It is simple prudence for the West to respond. We in Britain intend to do that to the best of our ability and at every level including the strategic.*"

The Soviet invasion of Afghanistan a few days later on December 27, 1979 had only strengthened her suspicion of the Soviet Union and her fears seem to have rubbed off on the country as a whole. When I landed in Britain in 1980, the country was in a state of hysterical paranoia expecting Russian soldiers to land on its soil any moment. TV channels aired both serious documentaries that appeared almost farcical, as well as light-hearted sitcoms depicting life in Britain after a Soviet invasion.

On the domestic front, as the prime minister of an increasingly multicultural nation, Margaret Thatcher failed to exude the benevolent statesman-like persona that one would expect. She came across as an imperious hawk, an impression that was more in keeping with a leader of the

Opposition than a prime minister. Most disconcerting was a sneering scowl that frequently made its appearance on her face. Added to this was her condescending tone of voice which broke into an irritating whine when overcome with strong emotion. In short she appeared like a headmistress lecturing her students.

Specifically, she failed to infuse any confidence in the immigrant population. She had already made her position clear on immigration in the run-up to the general election: she was dead opposed to it. In a TV interview for *Granada World in Action*in January 1978 she had said:

> "*Well now, look, let us try and start with a few figures as far as we know them, and I am the first to admit it is not easy to get clear figures from the Home Office about immigration, but there was a committee which looked at it and said that if we went on as we are then by the end of the century there would be four million people of the new Commonwealth or Pakistan here. Now, that is an awful lot and I think it means that people are really rather afraid that this country might be rather swamped by people with a different culture and, you know, the British character has done so much for democracy, for law and done so much throughout the world that if there is any fear that it might be swamped, people are going to react and be rather hostile to those coming in.*"

Her stand on immigration had been severely criticized by political leaders and prominent clergymen, but her remarks had found a favorable audience among a significant section of the electorate. Following the interview, the Tories surged ahead of Labour in opinion polls for the first time. Margaret Thatcher had successfully played the immigration card, a strategy that would eventually carry her to victory.

So, when she did actually become prime minister, there was a definite sense of trepidation in the Asian immigrant community and Mrs. Thatcher did little to allay those fears. In fact her utterances and uncompromising attitude increased the distrust. A particularly telling TV interview comes to mind.

At that time there were no TV channels that catered exclusively to the South Asian community. The only South Asian program was a variety show that was broadcast by BBC on Sunday mornings. It was a short presentation that lasted no more than half an hour and consisted of a news segment that narrated events from the subcontinent that were a week old, local happenings and a popular Hindi song which acted as the finale. Nazia Hassan's *Aap Jaisa Koi Meri Zindagi Mein Aaye*was the rage during those days and was invariably the curtain closer of this show. Putting all this together and serving as an anchor for this variety program was an aging, grandfatherly Asian gentleman who must have been an inhabitant of Britain for at least 30 years. He was the face of the Asian community on British TV.

On one of these shows this elderly gentleman happened to interview Margaret Thatcher. Throughout the interview the gentle and self-effacing anchor made a genuine and sincere effort to reach out to Margaret Thatcher, trying to extract some sort of assurance from her for the Asians in Britain. But all his pleading for Asians to be included in Margaret Thatcher's vision of a future UK came to naught; they hit a stone wall. The "Iron Lady" did not wilt or exhibit any compassion. Although she did not say it in so many words, her steely composure said it all:

immigrants were not welcome under her regime.

The anchor's crestfallen face at the end of the interview embodied the plight of the Asian in Britain then: permanent rejection from British society after having spent a lifetime in that country.

To be fair, my colleagues who never made it across the pond and who currently live in Britain tell me that the race situation in Britain did improve greatly over the next three decades leading to a greater acceptance of Asians into the mainstream of British life during the late 90s and the first decade of the twenty-first century. Nevertheless, racism among the British is a deep-seated trait; it may be transiently lost in the hurly-burly environment of a rapid-paced globalized universe but is rarely far from the surface, as a young immigrant Indian student who moved to a welcoming Britain in 2005 discovers five years later in 2010. Read this excerpt from the Indian online news portal, Rediff:

> "*The country I moved to in 2005 as a student was not a rainbow nation where people of each color stuck to their own. It was a veritable melting pot where, largely, people of different races intermingled quite comfortably.... There was recognition in the mainstream that the definition of what it meant to be British had changed, and Britain was all the richer for it.*
>
> *However, a lot appears to have changed over the past few years....*
>
> *The country I live in in 2010 still remains a melting pot. However, there is a palpable change in the atmosphere. The polemical headlines on Britain's right-wing tabloids, never renowned for*

their xenophilia, have grown evermore hostile towards immigrants, particularly those of Asian and African extraction. Almost every article on immigration features images of black and brown people, preferably those wearing burqas.

But what is more worrying than the tabloid headlines themselves is the alarming rapidity with which British political parties have given up any pretence to having any ideology beyond the appeasement of Middle England and its favorite tabloids. Additionally, all three political parties require a scapegoat to blame for the multiple failures of the neo-liberal economic principles they have championed for the past several years. And what better scapegoat can one wish for than non-white immigrants, who comprise a mere 8 percent of the population?

Is today's multicultural Britain likely to be burnt in the raging fires of an economy in crisis, presided over by a hard-line government that wishes to cover for its sins by whipping up a xenophobic frenzy? Will the Britain I saw in 2005 – where I almost immediately felt at home – survive into 2015?"

("Is Multicultural Britain Dead?" SiddhuWarrier, *Rediff*, December 3, 2010)

CHAPTER TEN

A Challenging Assignment and My First Liver Biopsy

I instructed Mr. Weatherby to hold his breath, a directive that would decrease any respiratory shifting of the liver, minimizing the possibility of a tear. And in one swift movement I thrust the needle into his liver and pulled it back almost instantaneously, trapping a piece of his liver in the needle notch in the process. Mr. Weatherby winced and then relaxed. The procedure was over. It had taken exactly three seconds.

Next stop Walsall and, the train chugged along. Despite a sense of crippling dejection at the slow progress of my career, I tried to infuse some levity into my life by comparing my itinerant plight to that of a slow passenger train. And in this journey, my next stop was Walsall.

My trip to Walsall did not carry with it even the hope of transient stability that a confirmed locum position offers; it was merely for an interview, a trek that may come to naught, leaving me in a state of limbo with no place to go and no job to do. Therefore it was with mixed feelings that I made this journey.

Walsall is a fair-sized industrial town with a population close to 200,000 located to the northwest of Birmingham. However I was totally oblivious of the size or significance of this town at that time. My stay in the UK consisted of direct trips from either the bus stand or train station to hospital premises and back. I saw or noticed precious little of the outside world; the same with Walsall.

There was one piece of information about the demographic distribution of Walsall that became evident to me as I looked around. The town had a fair sprinkling of Asians and mirrored the concentration of Asians around the Birmingham area. Today Asians make up about 14 percent of the population here compared to a national average of 4 percent.

My first recollection of Walsall is my interview at Manor Hospital. It did bother me a little that this interview was for the position of a house officer, a rank that was one rung below my level of training. The redeeming feature however was that it was a permanent job, a post that had a tenure of six months. Equating six months with permanency would certainly make anyone burst out with laughter, but for a physician accustomed to locum positions that lasted for just a few days or weeks, six months was like an eternity that conferred some degree of stability to one's existence.

In addition to myself, there were three other candidates vying for the position: a Pakistani, an Arab and another young physician whose nationality I could not determine. As we waited to be called in, we made small talk with each other in an attempt to soothe the butterflies in our respective bellies. Each interview lasted about 15 minutes. Finally my turn came. I was the last of the four to be interviewed.

Having been to umpteen interviews in a short span of six months, I thought of myself as a hardened professional when it came to facing the interview board. However in this instance I was a little more anxious than usual, probably because it was my first interview for a regular job. The panel consisted of three consultant physicians and to my surprise, one of them was Indian. To find an Indian physician, that too a consultant, in general medicine was rare. The Indian consultant was Dr Talwalkar, whom I would come to know better in the next few days.

The interview followed the same pattern: a review of my résumé, some questions regarding my previous job and finally the million dollar question that was a constant fixture at all interviews: Did I plan to settle in Britain or go back to India?

The other option of moving to the US was usually not broached as it constituted an affront to British sensibilities: it indicated that the US was better than Britain and for a people who had still not become accustomed to their status as an ex-colonial power, this was hard to digest.

The answer to the question constituted a Hobson's choice: a tails-you-lose-heads-he-wins situation. With the growing antipathy towards immigrants in Britain a desire to stay back was frowned upon and was certainly not the right option. And in case you answered that you would like to go back to your country you were immediately confronted with the following riposte: Why should we expend our resources and train you if you are going to go back and not be of use to us?

Of the two the second choice was less controversial and less likely to evoke a harsh response and I settled for that on most occasions.

The interview over, we waited expectantly for the outcome. Eventually the administrator, a smartly-suited young gentleman emerged from the interview room, pointed to the physician of unknown nationality and escorted him inside, an indication that he was the chosen one. For the rest us it was a signal to pack up, hand in our travel expense voucher and make ourselves scarce. But the administrator turned to the rest of us and instructed us not to leave. There was still some unfinished business. Two locum positions had to be filled: a four-week locum for a house officer and a locum of the same duration for a registrar.

I was called in next. I walked in expecting to be offered the house officer locum that I would have gladly accepted. So when Dr Talwalkar asked me whether I was willing to function as a locum registrar, I was taken aback. A rash of questions swirled through my mind in an instant. Was I capable of handling this enhanced responsibility? Did I have the requisite experience? All my experience in general medicine in the UK had been at the house officer level. This meant an upgrade to two rungs higher. And if I did refuse the offer what were my other choices? I really didn't have any.

Why not accept this job, I told myself. I had nothing to lose. Additionally, it would net me a few extra pounds that

I could surely use. Mustering up all my courage I mouthed a definitive yes opening up another chapter in my career in the UK that would be part challenging and part daunting.

My first challenge confronted me the moment I walked in to the medical unit the next morning to take charge. Waiting to receive me was my house officer, Dr Ibrahim Khan, a young, affable Pakistani physician. The fact that Dr Khan hailed from Pakistan, a country that I was not particularly fond of, was not what unsettled me. It was his inexperienced status: he too was a locum like myself and had started his tenure a day earlier. A new position that I had hesitatingly accepted as it demanded a higher level of expertise and responsibility suddenly became even more daunting by the added encumbrance of over-seeing another greenhorn. However my initial concerns were overcome by Dr Talwalkar, my consultant. He more than made up for the handicap that Dr Khan posed to me. Dr Talwalkar was by nature a kind individual. He was soft-spoken, mild and not in the least intimidating as most consultants are prone to be. He guided me through this difficult period with practical advice and sound medical education exhibiting extraordinary patience and understanding. I cannot thank him enough for that.

Dr Talwalkar hailed from the western Indian state of Gujarat and had emigrated to the UK in the early 60s. He was one of those rare Indian consultants that you came across in the UK at that time. Elevation to the post of a consultant for an Indian was not based purely on professional merit. There was a social element built into it. Those who became consultants invariably had wives of British extraction, an unwritten prerequisite to be a consultant. Dr Talwalkar too had a British wife.

Somehow I felt that marrying a Britisher was not purely a personal choice for these individuals. It appeared to have a broader intent and significance. In addition to the professional advantage, there appeared to be a psychological angle to it. Was it a subconscious effort to merge in with the mainstream of British life and blunt the overt racism that one encountered, I wondered. And Indians who married British women appeared to develop a distinct personality complex characterized by an exaggerated anti-Indian undercurrent. It was not unusual to come across these individuals holding forth on India's backwardness or make caustic remarks about Indians. However Dr Talwalkar did not belong to this ilk. He still preserved a soft corner for fellow Indians.

Dr Talwalkar, by virtue of having worked at Manor Hospital for a long time, had been anointed as the senior consultant, a position of some honor. But this had not gone down too well with the other consultants in the hospital who all happened to be British. Extremely vocal about this was Dr Taggart, who was much younger than Dr Talwalkar, but who just could not stomach the idea of being subordinate to Dr Talwalkar. He rarely passed up an opportunity to express his displeasure. Once I heard him complaining to a colleague, "We brought these Indians here to work for us, not to rule us."

Biopsy is a word with a Greek origin and comes from *bios*meaning life and *opsis*which means "to see." In medical terms this refers to a diagnostic study in which a piece of tissue from the diseased organ is obtained for further microscopic examination. This tissue can be obtained by simply cutting out a piece of the skin in dermatological conditions or using a needle to access internal organs like the liver or kidney. Less commonly an operation may be required to acquire the required tissue.

It was my second day at Walsall when I encountered my first practical challenge. As I sat in the doctors' lounge going over my schedule for the next day, I noticed with some degree of trepidation a liver biopsy listed against my name. I had performed a fair number of liver biopsies back in India and was technically competent to perform the procedure, but the new location and the thought of unfamiliar instruments added a degree of uncertainty to the process.

Every medical procedure has an inherent risk of complication that does not strictly correlate at all times with the experience or level of training of the operator. Today I repeatedly tell medical students that medicine is not a perfect science. In medicine, 2 plus 2 does not always translate into 4; it can be 3 or 5. Complications are known to occur even at the hands of physicians who have been in practice for a lifetime and who have performed thousands of similar procedures; hence my concern.

As I mulled over the complications of a liver biopsy, I chanced to notice Dr Gopalkrishnan, an Indian physician whom I had met the previous day. Like me, he hailed from the southern part of India and I felt he was a kindred spirit, realizing only later that this was a mistake. He was a registrar on Dr Taggart's unit and had been working in Walsall for over a year. I approached him for support seeking some sort of a mental reassurance rather than any definite physical assistance, only to be rebuffed with the retort that one should not accept responsibilities that one could not handle. Ironically, this negative response firmed my resolve and I approached the procedure the next day with added confidence. I *had* to succeed.

The liver is a reddish-brown organ that weighs about 3 pounds and is triangular in shape. It occupies a recess in the right upper quadrant of the abdomen underneath the overhanging rib cage. Two things make a liver biopsy a risky procedure. The liver being a highly vascular organ is more likely to bleed in the event of any injury. Post-procedure bleeding is the most serious and most dreaded complication of a liver biopsy. Fortunately, when properly performed less than 1 percent of patients develop significant bleeding. This statistic though reassuring when viewed in broad terms is hardly comforting in the face of a real complication. A colleague of mine rightly pointed out that when a complication does occur it amounts to 100 percent for the patient and seems like 100 percent for the physician as well.

Second, a liver biopsy done in the traditional fashion is what one would call a "blind procedure": the physician does not actually see the organ but assumes that the organ is where he is inserting his needle or biopsy device. There have been instances where the needle has been inadvertently inserted into the lung or the kidney. To overcome such risks, liver biopsies nowadays are increasingly performed under the guidance of a CT scan which allows for visualization of the liver prior to inserting the needle. Death from a liver biopsy, though always a possibility, is very rare in present times.

The liver biopsy was scheduled for 9 in the morning. I walked briskly into the minor operating room or OR as it is called, trying to hide my anxiety, and scanned the pages of the patient's medical record to acquaint myself with his history. Mr. Weatherby, the patient, was a Caucasian gentleman in his mid-50s who had been experiencing intermittent bouts of fever coupled with progressive fatigue for the previous two months. Blood tests and other investigations had failed to come up with an answer. The only abnormality noted was in his liver function tests. Hence, the liver biopsy.

I spent a good 15 minutes explaining to Mr Weatherby the details of the procedure including its potential risks and benefits. At the end of my mini-lecture he nodded his prompt assent. There was no extensive interrogation of my medical background or questions about the number of liver biopsies that I had done, something that I consistently encounter nowadays. That was an era in which trust was the only bond that cemented a physician and his patient with both sides sincerely honoring the abstract commitment. Formal printed consents were not even heard of in those times.

My first task was to locate the position of the liver. For that I tentatively tapped the area in-between his lower ribs on their lateral aspect with my fingers, an action that is referred to in medical jargon as percussion, to locate an area of dullness that would indicate the position of the liver. I marked that area with an "X" sign. After cleaning the surrounding area with iodine to get rid of any bacteria residing on the skin surface I proceeded to cover it with a sterile blue drape that had a small hole in the center through which the "X" mark showed: the site through which I would insert my needle.

The next step involved numbing the area with a local anesthetic and using a scalpel (a knife) to make a small cut which would provide an entry site for my biopsy needle. I eyed the biopsy needle lying on the table by my side nervously. It was of the Tru-cut variety, a modern version of the archaic one that I was used to in India. The Tru-cut device consists of a needle bearing a notch close to its tip sheathed in an outer cover. On closer examination, I was reassured to note that the design was essentially similar to the older model. The principle of usage was also going to be the same.

Mustering up all my confidence I slowly inserted the needle through the cut that I had made until I felt the resistance of the liver edge. There is no definite gauge as to when this point is reached. It is all about "feel." The last and most crucial aspect of the test entails close cooperation between the patient and physician. I instructed Mr Weatherby to hold his breath, a directive that would decrease any respiratory shifting of the liver, minimizing the possibility of a tear. And in one swift movement I thrust the needle into his liver and pulled it back almost instantaneously, trapping a piece of his liver in the needle notch in the process. Mr. Weatherby winced and then relaxed. The procedure was over. It had taken exactly three seconds.

The core of liver tissue that I had obtained was nearly 15 mm long, adequate to prevent the pathologist from complaining of paucity of tissue.

For the next six hours, I confined Mr. Weatherby to the bed, advising him to lie on his right side, and instructed the nurse to monitor his pulse and blood pressure every 15 minutes. Mr. Weatherby suffered no complication and went home that evening. I heaved a huge sigh of relief.

About a week into my new job I was called to the emergency room one night to treat a teenager who had been brought in unconscious. From his looks - purple-colored hair, patched up jeans and the myriad tattoos that dotted his arms and torso - I gathered he belonged to the genre of wayward unemployed youth that were common in Britain of the 80s. I shook him vigorously trying to elicit a response, but to no avail. The nurse who had triaged him informed me that he had a low blood pressure. His pulse was barely palpable and he was breathing laboriously and slowly with prolonged pauses that threatened to cease any moment.

For a moment I suffered a bout of mental paralysis not knowing what was wrong with the young lad or what to do. I hastily ran through a gamut of differential diagnoses that could explain his predicament. When I pulled open his eyelids to look at his pupils I found my answer: his pupils were constricted or what we physicians call pinpoint, a definite sign of heroin overdose. I quickly scanned his arms for needle tracks that confirmed my suspicion.

I asked the nurse for a dose of naloxone, which is an antidote to heroin, and promptly injected it into the intravenous tubing that ran into his arm. The response was almost instantaneous. The teenager opened his eyes, lazily surveyed the room and mumbled something incoherently. A few minutes later he was making sensible conversation with all the personnel in the emergency room. Inwardly, I congratulated myself on my competence and success.

Thirty minutes later, after making sure that he was fully awake, I took leave. No sooner had I reached the other end of the emergency ward than I heard the nurse call out to me desperately. I rushed back to find the patient lapsing back into unconsciousness. I ordered another dose of naloxone which transiently reversed his condition. But this cycle kept repeating itself and I spent the entire night by his bedside, dosing him repeatedly with naloxone to keep him awake and alive. Finally I decided to admit him to the intensive care unit as opposed to a regular ward using my prerogative as a registrar.

Intensive care beds are scarce and an object of contention between competing services. As a registrar I was expected to decide which patients required admission to the hospital and to designate the specific units their conditions warranted. What I had considered to be an astute decision the night before was not dittoed by Dr Talwalkar the next morning. As I began the routine daily task of reviewing the previous night's admissions I saw a deep frown cloud Dr Talwalkar's face. Patients indulging in drug abuse are looked upon as a nuisance as they detract from other patients more worthy of medical attention. Therefore to "waste" an intensive care bed on a case of heroin overdose did not appear appropriate to him. However, after a detailed presentation of the case, which involved an event-by-event recall of the previous night, Dr Talwalkar did appreciate my point of view.

The doctors' residence in Walsall had a common kitchen that was kept well stocked by non-physician spouses, a fair number of whom happened to be from India. It was in this hallowed spot that I was initiated into the ritual of cooking. Until then I was a complete novice to this field. My only foray into the intricate process of food preparation had been a botched effort during a Boy Scout outing when I was 14. An attempt to prepare a spiced Indian version of spaghetti turned out to be an unmitigated disaster. Instead of a pleasant-smelling and enticing dish, the end product had been a glob of mashed spaghetti with an excessive amount of green Indian jalapenos that made its ingestion almost impossible. Needless to say, the scout master asked me to discard the preparation.

After months of bland English food I was tempted to try my hand at cooking once more. The timing was appropriate. It was a long weekend and most residents were away. I had the kitchen all to myself and lots of time to kill. It was an ideal opportunity for some culinary adventuring.

I kept the menu simple: plain rice and something to go with it. Cooking rice was the easy part. I had seen my mother do it a thousand times. All you had to do was to wash the grains of rice under a running faucet, place one measure of the washed rice along with two measures of water in a covered metal container and allow it to cook for approximately 30 minutes.

The "something to go with it" was the difficult part. I toyed with the idea of making some dal, the spiced lentil soup-like preparation that is usually served with rice, but soon dismissed the idea. I didn't know the exact recipe and couldn't decide which of the three different lentils arrayed on the kitchen shelf to use.

Eventually I settled for a vegetable curry with potatoes and onions. It is remarkable how a simple act of slicing an onion can become an onerous task when one doesn't know how. Every time I tried to get the onion to take the shape of those uniformly cut pieces similar to the ones in my mother's curries, the errant half-cut bulb slipped away from underneath the knife. Months later a female colleague of mine pointed out my mistake and taught me the art of cutting an onion: the half-cut bulb needs to be placed with its flat surface facing the cutting board and not the other way around as I was trying to do. After a few botched attempts, I was finally able to get the potatoes and onions into suitably small pieces that were appropriate for cooking.

Next I proceeded to pour some vegetable oil along with a spoonful of mustard seeds into a cooking pot and allowed it to warm up. When the mustard seeds began to pop, indicating that the oil had reached the required temperature, I added the potatoes and onions and deftly mixed them together with a tablespoon. Just as I was patting myself on my back for the professional manner in which I was handling this cooking adventure I realized that I had forgotten the most important part of a curry preparation: the addition of herbs and spices, better known as "masalas."

With a sense of bewilderment I eyed the array of tiny bottles lining the shelf. There were umpteen of them, each containing a differently colored powder: bright yellow, angry red and plain gray to describe a few. Without knowing exactly what each powder was, I added a pinch from the first three bottles in no specific order and stirred them into the onion-potato mixture. Finally I emptied a cup of water into the simmering concoction and allowed it to cook for about 30 minutes.

The smell emanating from the brown-colored stew brewing in the pot was appetizing. I scooped up some of this curry in a ladle and deposited it beside the small mound of cooked rice spread out on a porcelain plate and sat down to savor my first self-prepared meal. Discarding all formalities, I did away with the use of any fork or spoon and used my clean, washed hands (Indians ritualistically wash their hands before sitting down for a meal) to mix the rice and curry together as I was used to in India.

The first morsel of this mixture to hit my palate was heavenly. The tantalizing tingling of Indian spices and the familiar feel of Indian cooked rice exploded my taste buds with excitement. Having been famished for Indian food for over six months this meal seemed to me like a feast fit for a king. Twenty years later even after frequenting the best Indian restaurants in different parts of the world, I still treasure the memory and taste of that meager lunch.

Walsall proved to be lucky for me. My stint as a locum registrar shored up my resume and gave me the break that I was waiting for.

Part Two

Relative Stability

CHAPTER ELEVEN

A Permanent Job at Last

South Shields? It may well have been Timbuktu. I had never heard of it before, and no clue where it was. But South Shields was where destiny took me in the early months of 1981.

Applying for a locum position was essentially a random exercise, a hit-or-miss proposition that was pursued with no preferences. You applied en masse for all the locum positions that were listed in that week's *BMJ,* because you never knew which would be your lucky one.So, considerations such as north, south, east or west; urban or rural; Scotland, England or Wales; Stoke-on-Trent, Turnbridge Wells or Barnsley, were totally irrelevant.

Only after you landed the job did you worry about pertinent details like the latitude and the longitude of the place and how to get there. South Shields? It may well have been Timbuktu. I had no clue where it was and had never heard of it before. But South Shields was where destiny took me in the early months of 1981.

South Shields according to the map (I had to make a special trip to the library to ascertain its bearings; mind you there was no Internet then) was a town located in the northeast of England close to the Scottish border and in a county with a strange name: Tyne and Wear.

"South Shields, South Shields, South Shields....?" the wispy old bespectacled clerk behind the ticketing counter muttered under his breath as he tried to answer my query.

He leafed through some dog-eared manuals on his cluttered desk, glanced at an officious board hanging on the wall behind him and declared," There is no direct train to South Shields. You can take the 7.03 from Birmingham New Street to Newcastle and switch to a local train," he advised me.

The 7.03 arrived on the dot like most British trains. I found a window seat and made myself comfortable. I spent the journey pondering over the merits and demerits of the job that awaited me. I was both excited and apprehensive. Excited because it was the longest job offer that I had received till then, a whole four and half months, from mid-March to the end of July. Apprehensive because it was a locum position in chest medicine. Chest medicine was an unattractive and less desirable subspecialty of general medicine. It dealt with the treatment of infectious diseases such as tuberculosis and most young British physicians looked down upon it. Would it dampen my future prospects, I wondered.

But then I was in no position to be choosy. I consoled myself with the fact that as chest medicine was classified under the broad umbrella of general medicine, it would be okay. Moreover, the administrator who had offered me this job, had dangled a carrot in front of me: there was a strong possibility that I would be asked to continue in the regular position that would become available after August 1.

It was almost noon when the train pulled into Newcastle-upon-Tyne. The next leg of my journey involved a short stint onboard a local train. Local trains tended to be less crowded than the ones on the main thoroughfare and the one from Newcastle to South Shields was no different. The compartments were empty for the greater part save for a lone passenger here and there. After my unpleasant encounter with skinheads in a London commuter train, I was careful to avoid sparsely populated areas lest I met the same fate again. I picked a compartment that was partially full, chose a seat near the door ready for an emergency exit if conditions so warranted and settled down with a book to read.

The local train lumbered past stations that were typically English-sounding, like Gateshead, and others that just didn't fit any description, like Jarrow and Tyne Dock. The countryside was unappealing - swaths of barren land and quite a few defunct dock yards. The deserted but expansive dockyards were tell-tale signs of the region's notable past as well as its unenviable present. These abandoned dockyards along with the partially decrepit houses that lined the streets completed a depressing picture of general penury.

Later, I would learn that South Shields had once been a prestigious shipping hub because of its strategic location at the point where the River Tyne meets the North Sea. But with the decline of the shipping industry post World War II, the town had receded into obscurity losing both its importance as well as its means of sustenance. The death of the shipping industry had a domino effect, leading to the closure of local collieries, the other main source of employment that depended heavily on the coal-driven ships for their growth.

The net result was rampant unemployment: jobs were scarce to come by in South Shields and the area had the highest unemployment rate in all of Great Britain. Bad times had chipped away its identity and reduced it to nothing more than a nondescript suburb of Newcastle-upon-Tyne located 10 miles away.

The dismal picture of ubiquitous poverty in the South Shields area unfolding before my eyes through the train window set me brooding again about my decisions and the future.

Once again, I had to shake myself out of this ominous foreboding by reminding myself that this was only a stepping stone and not my final destination.

The South Shields hospital complex consisted of old, brick-faced, yet sturdy buildings spaciously dispersed over an expansive area of land near the outskirts of the town. Here and there, one came across a modern structure with a vinyl exterior that stood out like a sore thumb, but also reminded you how ancient the other buildings were.

The entrance led you up a tarred pathway to the main hospital building, an archaic but impressive-looking edifice that must have been at least a hundred years old. It was shaped like a capital H with annexes on either side linked together by a central wing that housed the administrative offices.

On your immediate right before you reached the main hospital was a boxy looking building, pedestrian in appearance compared to the majestic looking hospital building, despite being a recent addition. This was the doctors' quarters which would become my residence a few months later. Adjoining the modern doctors' residence was a quaint little cottage that was architecturally more esthetic. The cottage had a circular façade with a sharply pointed roof like the ones I had seen in fairy tale books. Inside, at the ground level, one encountered a doctors' lounge and an ample sized kitchenette; on the upper level were a couple of boarding rooms which were temporary residences meant for locums. One of these rooms was to be mine.

The lounge was a common meeting place for all physicians: we congregated there during lunch hours, at the end of a hard day's work or whenever we felt like we needed a brief respite from our daily chores. The atmosphere in the lounge was relaxed and leisurely with a pervading sense of camaraderie. It was here that we young physicians exchanged our professional travails, discussed politics, browsed through newspapers and prepared tea and coffee for one another. At that time we had no omnipresent coffee makers that brewed coffee 24/7. Coffee was prepared the old-fashioned way by boiling water in an aluminum kettle and could be a cumbersome process at times, especially if your previous colleague had misplaced the matchbox necessary to light the gas burner. Yet it was an unwritten rule that while preparing a cup for yourself you made coffee for everyone else present in the lounge regardless of your familiarity with them.

This tradition, apart from being a polite gesture, came in handy for other subtle machinations. For example it presented the perfect opportunity to strike up a conversation with the pretty little house officer from obstetrics and gynecology you had encountered on the wards the day before and were dying to talk to. These hospital lounges were the beginning point for many romantic dalliances, some transient and some permanent.

Facing this cottage was a grotesque building that appeared almost deserted. No one ever seemed to enter it, and for a long time, I did not know what it was. Later I would learn that it was the hospital morgue.

The hospital complex was demarcated on one side by a brick wall that ran along Harton Lane. Harton Lane was not a busy street and did not see much traffic but was the main access route to the hospital. By the entrance was a conveniently located bus stop where brown and yellow public buses stopped every 15 minutes to allow neatly dressed little old ladies with hospital appointments to get off.

The other side of the hospital complex overlooked rows of corn fields that suggested that the hospital was located somewhere near the outskirts of the town. Whether this was actually so or not I never did confirm during my entire two-year stay in South Shields. Not once did I venture into the corn fields to explore the area around the hospital on foot.

When I look back, I am appalled at the lack of interest I exhibited in my surroundings and my pathetic mental lethargy. To some extent it reflected the state of my mind at that time. I was completely trapped in a dismal world of my own making; a world that was unconsciously restricted to hospitals and exams – little else mattered. I now realize how much I lost out in the process.

One of the things that I regret most about my sojourn in South Shields is not making use of its proximity to the rest of Europe. A mere seven-minute boat ride from South Shields was the International Ferry terminal. For a few pounds, one could hop aboard a ferry at 5 p.m. in the evening and alight in Amsterdam the following morning. A weekend trip across the channel was a common outing among my physician colleagues, something I never ventured to be a part of.

Whether this self-absorption was a personal quirk dictated by my specific circumstance or a national trait borne out of a defined way of life is hard to tell. V. S. Naipaul, the Nobel Prize–winning author, feels that such insular behavior is an inherent Indian attribute, a contention that he bolsters with a critical analysis of an excerpt from Mahatma Gandhi's *The Story of My Experiments with Truth* that pertains to the Mahatma's trip in 1888 from Bombay to Southampton. In his book, Mahatma Gandhi wrote:

> "*I sailed at last from Bombay on the 4th of September. I did not feel at all sea-sick. But as the days passed, I became fidgety. I felt shy even in speaking to the steward. I was quite unaccustomed to talking English, and except for Sgt. Mazumdar all the other passengers in the second saloon were English. I could not speak to them. For I could rarely follow their remarks when they came up to speak to me, and even when I understood I could not reply. I had to frame every sentence in my mind, before I could bring it out. I was innocent of the use of knives and forks and had not the boldness to inquire what dishes on the menu were free of meat, I therefore never took meals at table but always had them in my cabin, and they consisted principally of sweets and fruits which I had brought with me. Sgt. Mazumdar had no difficulty, and he mixed with*

> *everybody. He would move about freely on deck, while I hid myself in the càbin the whole day, only venturing up on deck when there were but few people. Sgt. Mazumdar kept pleading with me to associate with the passengers and to talk with them freely. He told me that lawyers should have a long tongue, and related to me his legal experiences. He advised me to take every possible opportunity of talking English, and not to mind making mistakes which were obviously unavoidable with a foreign tongue. But nothing could make me conquer my shyness....However, we reached Southampton, as far as I remember, on a Saturday. On the boat I had worn a black suit, the white flannel one, which my friends had got me, having been kept especially for wearing when I landed. I had thought that white clothes would suit me better when I stepped ashore, and therefore I did so in white flannels. Those were the last days of September, and I found I was the only person wearing such clothes.* "

(*The Story of My Experiments with Truth*, M. K. Gandhi)

Critiquing this description, in his book, *India: A Wounded Civilisation*, Naipaul comments:

> "*That is the voyage: an internal adventure of anxieties felt and food eaten, with not a word of anything seen or heard that did not directly affect the physical or mental well being of the writer. The inward concentration is fierce, the self-absorption complete. Southampton is lost in that embarrassment about the white flannels. The name*

of the port is mentioned once, and that is all, as though the name is description enough.... Though Gandhi spent three years in England, there is nothing in his autobiography about the climate or the season...and the next date he is precise about is the date of his departure.

No London building is described, no street, no room, no crowd, no public conveyance. The London of 1890, capital of the world – which must have been overwhelming to a young man from a small India town – has to be inferred from Gandhi's continuing internal disturbances, his embarrassments, his religious self-searching, his attempts at dressing correctly and learning English manners and, above all, his difficulties and occasional satisfaction with food."

CHAPTER TWELVE

South Shields: The Early Days

As we stood at the nurses' station exchanging glancing uncertainly at each other and looking more like lost schoolboys than full-fledged physicians, she realized our predicament and promptly reassured us that things were under control.

It was mid-March when I reached South Shields to start my new job. Old Man Winter was fading away making way for spring. My first winter in the Western hemisphere was coming to an end. I had managed to brave the harsh weather remarkably well despite never having been exposed to ice and snow before.

The barometer was gradually climbing and I no longer had to venture out covered head to toe in warm, suffocative clothing. I could do away with the monkey cap and the cumbersome scarf that I usually wrapped around my neck for added protection. At times when the wind chill factor made conditions even more unbearable, I used to unfold the scarf and pull it over my nose leaving only my eyes exposed and looking like a masked bandit. Neither was I too fond of the gloves that were indispensable for preventing my fingers from turning numb.

The sun now made its appearance more often and the days were getting longer. Trees were sprouting leaves, the grass was getting greener and the chirping of the birds was getting louder.

I was amazed at these distinct changes that marked the end of one season and the beginning of another. In the south of India where I hail from, it appeared that we had basically only two seasons: when it rained, and when it did not. The trees never showed such a remarkable transformation from being completely bereft of leaves in winter to having a full shock of leaves in summer.

Back home, daylight hours remained the same throughout the year with minor changes that were really not discernible and which did not affect any changes to our lifestyle. Moving the clocks forward in summer and back in fall was an alien concept to me and I found it rather amusing. I just could not understand how changing the hands on a clock would make any difference to one's pattern of working.

On my first day, I walked into the chest unit all excited and raring to go. Standing next to the nurses' station were two other physicians: a thirtyish Indian male clad in a white apron - the other SHO - and another middle-aged Indian, attired in a pin-stripe suit, who I rightly presumed was the Consultant. I strode up to them, introduced myself with a chirpy smile and remarked," I am the new SHO. Today is my first day."

To which the younger of the two physicians replied," Welcome. Today is my first day as well."

And even before I could comprehend his response, the Consultant chimed in, "Mine too."

An uncomfortable silence ensued. All of us froze as the implication of our statements sank in.

In Walsall, on my first day, I had to contend with one other colleague who was starting afresh. Here, the entire physician complement of the chest medicine team, including the consultant, was new. There was no departing physician to fill us in on the cases in the ward. To call such a situation unsettling was an understatement: it was overwhelming, with a definite potential for chaos and medical blunders. The anxiety that gripped the air was almost palpable at that moment.

Medical care is a 24/7/365 business in which transition of care is inevitable and constantly taking place at the end of a working day, at the start of a weekend, at the end of a month when rotations for residents and house officers change and, at the end of a tenure of a physician. Even during the course of a single day, transfer of medical care takes place at multiple times, at multiple points and between multiple levels of health-care providers when shifts change, when patients are moved from one part of the hospital to another (for instance, from the emergency room to the wards) and when in-patients undergo operations or procedures. Detailed communication with a clear emphasis on the critical aspects of each patient's medical problems is essential for good medical care and to prevent a patient "falling through the cracks," as physicians say.

"Hand off" is the newly coined term used for the process in which one physician or a team of physicians transfer care of a patient or patients to another. In those days, we didn't have a designated term to refer to this process. It was the absence of a departing physician to fill us in on the relevant history of the in-patients of the ward that made our group of new physicians nervous.

Today in the US, transition of care is becoming more streamlined and blunders related to it are becoming less common. In 2007 the Joint Commission for Accreditation of Hospitals sought to make the "hand-off" procedure a standardized entity by classifying it as a "Patient National Safety Goal." The Joint Commission is an organization which is responsible for accreditation of health care in the US. JCAHO, as it is commonly called, analyzed 3,000 "sentinel events" (a sentinel event is defined by the Joint Commission as any unanticipated event in a healthcare setting resulting in death or serious physical or psychological injury to a patient or patients, not related to the natural course of the patient's illness) for the period 1995 to 2004 and found that over two-thirds were caused by miscommunication and over half of these errors occurred during the "hand off" phase.

In the 80s, we were not privy to statistical data about the deleterious effects of improper hand off. Nevertheless we were aware that good communication was important for good medical care. A face-to-face hand–off was much more crucial during those times when we had no computers to store information, and medical documentation tended to be sketchy and unregulated. We relied heavily on the word of the head nurse of the unit who was usually well-informed and guided us appropriately.

Sister O'Connor, the head nurse of our chest unit was our savior on our first day. As we stood at the nurses' station exchanging glancing uncertainly at each other with blank faces and empty looks that flitted back and forth from one another, making us look and looking more like lost schoolboys than full-fledged physicians, she realized our predicament and promptly reassured us that things were under control.

"Most of them are stable. There are only a couple of sick patients. Let me take you around." she ventured.

Sister O'Connor was a wisp of a woman, barely 5 feet 2 inches tall and mildly built; she could not have weighed more than 120 pounds. But her voice, usually sweet and nice, could be ratcheted up to convey a commanding authority.

With professional efficiency she gathered her "forces" that included two other nurses and a couple of nursing students, and ordered one of them to bring out the "charts cart", a dilapidated trolley that carried several cardboard binders containing loose sheets of paper that passed for medical records in those days. She bade us follow her as she marched out of the nurses' station and into the ward.

The ward was a long capacious room with a ceiling that must have been at least 20 feet in height. It gave the appearance of a godown that had been converted into a hospital ward. On either side of this gigantic room were rows of beds, 12 on either side to be exact. There were no curtains or screens to offer even a degree of privacy to the patients: it was one large communal hall. The male and female sections of the ward were not separated by a proper divider: the cluster of rooms that formed the nursing station and special treatment areas acted as a barrier between the two.

Our train comprising three nurses, three physicians and a few straggling student nurses moved slowly down this hall pausing in front of each bed to familiarize ourselves with the patient's problem. Each patient encounter lasted anywhere between 20 to 40 minutes and consisted of a brief synopsis of the patient's history provided by Sister O'Connor followed, if required, by a limited physical examination of the concerned organ system. A couple of cases proved to be diagnostic dilemmas and we spent extra time debating the possible diagnoses and charting out a future course of action. By the time we were done with our rounds, it was well past 6 p.m. It had been a long day but a satisfying one. The uncertainty and anxiety that we had experienced in the morning had been replaced with a quiet confidence that comes with a knowledgeable assessment of a situation.

CHAPTER THIRTEEN

Facing a Life and Death Situation

Then holding the chest tube with one hand and the trocar firmly clenched in my other fist and with a prayer on my lips, I thrust the tube through the incision. Once I was sure the tube was in the pleural cavity, I removed the trocar gingerly, positioned the tube and swung around to look at the underwater seal that was connected to its other end. I could see bubbles of air making their way up to the surface of the water indicating the success of my procedure. I heaved a sigh of relief.

The extended locum position in South Shields gave me a sense of relative stability, a breather that allowed me to put my luggage down and heave a much-needed sigh of relief. I could now apply myself whole-heartedly to the care of my patients without worrying about where I would be going the following day or whether I would have a roof over my head at the end of the week.

Here in South Shields, I went to work with a little more confidence in myself and a little more enthusiasm than what I had demonstrated in my early days in the UK. The atmosphere in the unit was casual and friendly. Dr Anthony, my consultant and boss, was an unassuming, mild-mannered, soft-spoken gentleman who did not believe in keeping his subordinates on a tight leash. He trusted us - that is my colleague and I - to do our job. Sister O'Connor had no airs about her either and was quite different from the snobbish head nurses I had encountered in Birmingham. All in all it was a pleasant place to work.

Dr Anthony was also an Indian and more or less in the same boat as we were: he too was a locum appointee. Our shared temporary status may have been instrumental in helping us bond, and we got along well.

Dr Anthony hailed from the state of Kerala, a coastal province of southern India with a significant Christian population. Christianity in Kerala goes a long way back. In fact, the Christians of Kerala trace their roots to St Thomas, one of the original 12 disciples of Jesus Christ who is supposed to have landed in Kerala in AD 52 to spread the message of Christ. Subsequently, the discovery of a sea route to India by the Portuguese mariner Vasco da Gama in 1492 and the British colonization of India helped spread Christianity among the Hindu population of Kerala.

Today Christians constitute about 19 percent of the population in Kerala, enjoy considerable political clout and are extremely prosperous. However the community is split into several sects, one of which is the Syrian Christian community. The Syrian Christians claim to be the first Christians of Kerala who were converted to Christianity by

St Thomas. Despite obliterating their Hindu past, Syrian Christians never fail to stress that they are descendants of high-caste Namboodiri Brahmins of Kerala, attesting to the overwhelming influence of castes in Indian society.

Christians from Kerala have a strange custom of using Christian first names as last names. Surnames like Peter, Paul, Stephen, George and Anthony are extremely common. Dr Anthony was a Syrian Christian in his mid-40s, thickset at the waist and with thinning hair at the back of his head. He had come to Britain via the "Gulf." The "Gulf" is a collective term used by Indians to refer to the conglomeration of monarchies around the Persian Gulf and includes places like Dubai, Abu Dhabi and Sharjah. The discovery of oil in the early part of the twentieth century gave a fillip to the economy of this region, and the consequent demand for labor and other amenities that this economic boom generated proved to be a bonanza for the money-strapped countries of neighboring South Asia. Indians, Pakistanis, Sri Lankans and Bangladeshis flocked to the Gulf in droves.

Indian doctors were also a part of this "gold rush" to the Gulf. Nevertheless, for the educated class-conscious Indian of the post-independence era the Gulf was always one rung lower in the hierarchy: the US came first and the UK second. Dr Anthony's dream was no different. He had spent a few years in the Gulf, earned significant tax-free income, and had then decided to come to Britain.

In Britain his career had taken a checkered course but that was only to be expected. However he had been more fortunate than most other Indians, managing to land a senior registrar position and complete a four-year stint at that level. This is a precondition to become a consultant, something that few other Indians could achieve. That was where his career path had hit a roadblock. Promotion to the next level, that of a consultant, was next to impossible. He would have to make do with locum consultant positions like the one that he had presently.

"Rounding" is a ritual that is the cornerstone of teaching in medicine during which a senior physician imparts knowledge acquired through years of experience to medical students and residents by direct interaction with a patient. For a junior physician, rounds with a senior physician constitute the high point of a working day and is a learning experience that he or she looks forward to. So it is important for a senior physician to make rounds interesting and informative.

However, making rounds with Dr Anthony was a lackluster affair. He made no attempt to expand the scope of discussion by including other possibilities in the differential diagnosis or by suggesting alternative modes of treatment. Rounds were brief, monosyllabic at times and strictly restricted to pertinent problems. They were work rounds rather than teaching rounds and tended to be mundane.

In Britain and in India, which inherited a British system of education, rounds are traditionally conducted at the bedside. We stand by the bed of the patient, discuss the problems, speak to the patient and examine him or her as a team. It is an interactive process that includes the patient in the dialogue.

Contrastingly, rounds in the US are conducted within the confines of a conference room away from the patient with greater emphasis on the information derived from investigations such as X-rays and CT scans. Of late however there has been a tendency to introduce a bedside component to these teaching exercises.

Ironically the concept of bedside teaching first originated in the US. The legendary physician William Harvey Osler was the original champion of bedside rounds which soon became a tradition among other Western nations. Osler was such an ardent devotee of bedside teaching that he wished to be remembered as one who "brought medical students into the wards for bedside teaching." He is said to have remarked, "I desire no other epitaph than the statement that I taught medical students in the wards, as I regard this as by far the most useful and important work I have been called upon to do."

Stressing the importance of bedside teaching, Osler used to tell his students: "He who studies medicine without books sails an uncharted sea, but he who studies medicine without patients does not go to sea at all."

Beset with concerns of privacy and patient sensitivity, rounds in the US gradually shifted to the conference room. However these concerns seem to be unfounded as recent studies have shown.

One study published in the *New England Journal of Medicine* in 1997 conducted by researchers from Johns Hopkins Hospital indicated that patients found bedside rounds reassuring and comforting as long as they were conducted in understandable language free of medical jargon. In recent times attempts are being made to resurrect bedside rounds at least to some extent.

*****

Despite the lack of formal teaching from my consultant, day-to-day work did provide me with significant practical education. In addition, the lack of a subordinate intern and a supervising registrar in our unit made my colleague and me efficient workhorses and presented us with challenges that refined our cognitive skills, a task that usually fell on the registrar.

Being a medicine/chest unit it was natural for us to encounter patients with diseases of the lung. The bulk of our admissions was made up of patients suffering from asthma and chronic obstructive pulmonary disorder (COPD). On a normal working day we admitted anywhere between five and eight patients with these conditions to our ward.

Asthma and COPD are often clubbed together because the manner in which they present - shortness of breath – is similar. The basic pathology is a narrowing or transient spasm of the air tubes that carry air from the outside to our lungs; this results in resistance to air flow and shortness of breath. A physician can detect this narrowing by auscultating the lungs.

Auscultation is a medical term that simply means "to listen" and owes its origin to the Latin word "*auscultaire.*" It is the process by which a physician listens to sounds emanating from certain body organs like the heart, lungs and the gastrointestinal system, with a view to ascertaining their workings. When a physician places a stethoscope on your chest during a physical examination, he is auscultating your heart or lungs.

Physicians were not always fortunate to have a stethoscope which is a relatively new addition to the practice of medicine. For centuries physicians listened to the internal sounds of the body by directly applying their ears to the chest and abdomen, a process they referred to as direct auscultation.

The stethoscope was invented in the early 1800s by the French physician Rene Laennec and was a product of expediency, necessitated by the need to preserve the modesty of a young female patient. In 1819, Laennec wrote a book titled,*De l'Auscultation Médiate ou Traité du Diagnostic des Maladies des Poumons et du Coeur*which literally translated means, "On Mediate Auscultation or Treatise on the Diagnosis of the Diseases of the Lungs and Heart," in which he outlines the circumstances that led him to this invention:

> "*In 1816, I was consulted by a young woman laboring under general symptoms of diseased heart, and in whose case percussion and the application of the hand were of little avail on account of the great degree of fatness. The other method just mentioned [direct auscultation] being rendered inadmissible by the age and sex of the patient, I happened to recollect a simple and well-known fact in acoustics - the great distinctness with which we hear the scratch of a pin at one end of a piece of wood on applying our ear to the other. Immediately, on this suggestion, I rolled a quire of paper into a kind of cylinder and applied one end of it to the region of the heart and the other to my ear, and was not a little surprised and pleased to find that I could thereby perceive the action of the heart in a manner much more clear and distinct than I had ever been able to do by the immediate application of my ear.*"

Laennec's prototype consisted of a hollow wooden cylinder about a foot long which he dubbed as the stethoscope combining the Greek word *stethos*(chest) with the French word *scope*(to view). The stethoscope eventually underwent several modifications to reach the form that we see today.

Although the stethoscope remains the hallmark of a physician, hanging prominently around his neck, its utility today has diminished greatly, superseded by the accuracy of more sophisticated technology. For example, with the advent of modern investigative instruments such as the echocardiogram, the stethoscope has been relegated to the status of a poor cousin in cardiac conditions and can be arguably dispensed with. But asthma is one disease in which I am of the opinion that the stethoscope has not lost its utility: neither a chest X-ray nor a CT scan can tell a physician what he is looking for – the presence of airway obstruction that is causing the patient to have difficulty in breathing.

Years of practice train a physician to differentiate abnormal breath sounds from normal ones. In asthma and COPD, normal breath sounds are replaced with abnormal sounds called *rhonchi* which are low-pitched sounds that remotely resemble the sound of snoring. These rhonchi signify the narrowing of the airways and can be detected only with a stethoscope.

The difference between asthma and COPD is more circumstantial: asthma occurs in persons of all ages, most of whom are non-smokers, while COPD is classically a disease of smokers over 40 years of age. The initial treatment of both these conditions is the same. One needs to dilate or open up the air tubes called bronchioles with medication. The treatment of even such a simple and widespread disease like asthma underlines the vast difference in medical facilities that exist between developed and underdeveloped nations. In the UK the first line of treatment involved the use of a nebulizer, a device that converts liquid medication into a fine aerosolized mist delivered directly to the bronchioles by means of compressed air without the need for painful injections. No needles, no syringes. The result is instantaneous and dramatic most of the time.

However, the only drugs available to us in India in those days were epinephrine and aminophylline, which were given via injections, one subcutaneously and the other intravenously. Disposable needles and syringes were unheard of. Syringes and needles were cleaned by dropping them into a cauldron of boiling water and wiping them dry with a hot towel fished out of the same container. Availability of oxygen was unpredictable. In fact in the rural health center that I was posted to during my internship, we went through long periods of oxygen shortage, so much so that whenever an asthma patient arrived I would pray fervently that he or she would respond promptly to subcutaneous epinephrine and would not require the use of oxygen. Epinephrine and aminophylline have now become almost obsolete in the treatment of asthma.

The most challenging situation that I encountered during my early days at South Shields was a case of pneumothorax. A pneumothorax is a physician's emergency, a condition which, if not treated promptly, can prove fatal. To understand the danger posed by this condition, one needs to know a little bit about the anatomy of the lungs. Each lung in our body is encased in a double-layered protective airtight covering called the pleura which protects the lung from the surrounding structures in the chest. The space between the two layers is called the pleural cavity, which contains minimal fluid and is normally collapsed with absolutely no air. Pneumothorax is a clinical condition in which air seeps into the pleural cavity by breaching the pleura. The break in the lining functions like a one-way valve allowing air to enter the pleural cavity but prevents it from escaping so that with every breath one takes the pleural cavity gets bigger and bigger. With the space in the chest being limited this expansion of the pleural cavity squeezes the lung and makes the life-sustaining act of breathing difficult.

A pneumothorax can complicate the course of diseases like COPD or it can be the result of an injury to the chest wall caused by a gunshot or a stab wound. Often it occurs without any apparent cause, a condition called spontaneous pneumothorax. That was what Derek had. Spontaneous pneumothorax is commonly seen in young male patients between the ages of 20 and 40.

Derek was 22 years of age, a local South Shields lad. He had woken up one Saturday morning and had been going about his morning routine when he started experiencing some breathing difficulty. At first he paid little attention to it hoping that it would pass. But when it persisted he became concerned and called an ambulance to take him to the hospital. A chest X-ray detected a pneumothorax and he was promptly transferred to our unit for treatment.

When I said earlier that this was a challenging situation it was not an overstatement. I knew the theory that it entailed: one had to insert a tube from the outside into the pleural cavity to provide access for the air to escape. I had seen some of my senior colleagues managing such cases. I had never treated a patient with a pneumothorax before.

The scenario that a pneumothorax presents is dramatic and my encounter with Derek was no different. When I walked into the room I found Derek sitting upright on the bed tightly clutching the rails. He was gasping for breath and his speech was barely audible, consisting of truncated phrases that came out in short bursts. He was sweating profusely from head to foot as he begged me to help him. I could see his condition deteriorating rapidly before my eyes; each breath seemed more labored than the previous one with every muscle in his neck stretching itself to overcome this deficiency of oxygen. The image was frightening.

For a moment I was transfixed, completely overwhelmed by the situation at hand. Then I felt Susan's hand nudge me. Susan was one of the charge nurses, a dignified young woman in her late 20s who spoke little, yet exuded a strong sense of warmth and confidence.

"You can do it, doctor," she exhorted me pushing the chest tube kit in front of me. I sized up the kit, jerked myself out of my trance and got down to work. Every second was important. I had no time to lose. The chest X-ray hanging on the view box told me that the pneumothorax was on the right side. I marked out the site through which I would insert the tube – between the fourth and fifth ribs along the side of the chest – and proceeded to make a one-inch incision with a scalpel (a small knife). Then holding the chest tube with one hand and the trocar firmly clenched in my other fist and with a prayer on my lips, I thrust the tube through the incision. Once I was sure the tube was in the pleural cavity I removed the trocar gingerly, positioned the tube and swung around to look at the underwater seal that was connected to its other end. I could see bubbles of air making their way up to the surface of the water indicating the success of my procedure. I heaved a sigh of relief.

When I turned to face Derek I saw a different person: his breathing was more normal, his face was free of agony and his incipient smile seemed to say thank you. I listened to his lungs with my stethoscope to ensure that adequate air was entering the lungs, ordered a chest X-ray to confirm the position of the tube and quickly walked out of the room. I didn't want Derek to see the perspiration on my face. Once outside I pulled out a handkerchief from my pocket, wiped off the beads of sweat trickling down my forehead and sat down on a chair to calm my racing heart.

While we encountered cases of asthma and COPD in the wards, the out-patient clinic was a parade of aging shipyard workers suffering from asbestosis-related lung problems. This was to be expected considering South Shields' past as the hub of the shipping industry. In fact on any given day more than half the patients presenting to the clinic suffered from asbestosis.

Asbestos is a mineral made up of silicon and oxygen. The word asbestos is derived from the Greek language and means "inextinguishable" or "indestructible." Because of its sturdy nature, asbestos found use initially in a variety of industries: shipping, automobile and construction.

However, asbestos becomes deadly when it is released into the air during manufacture or during installation of completed products. Decay of asbestos-containing products may also contribute to this process. Once inhaled, asbestos fibers lodge themselves in the lung tissue, provoke an inflammatory response

and produce scarring of the lung tissue rendering it functionless, a condition called asbestosis. This damage is easily visible in a simple chest X-ray. Instead of the translucent appearance of the lung seen in healthy individuals one saw patches of opaque areas that denoted fibrosis (medical term for simple scarring). When one combined this picture with the patient's difficulty in breathing and his former occupation as a shipyard worker, the diagnosis was not difficult to make.

But our biggest concern and mission was to detect early signs of cancer in these patients. Cancer was one of the dreaded complications of asbestosis. Any change in the patient's weight, a worsening of symptoms and new findings in the patient's chest X-ray made us nervous. One particular ominous sign was a pleural effusion or a collection of fluid in the lining of the lungs which we refer to as the pleura. A pleural effusion heralded its presence as a continuous white haziness occupying the lower part of the lung, the extent of the lung obscured indicating the amount of the fluid present. Some effusions were large enough to cover the entire lung.

It was almost inevitable that long term shipyard workers developed asbestosis. A study conducted by the Mount Sinai Medical Center in New York found that close to 90 percent of workers who had worked 20 years or more in the shipping industry were liable to develop asbestos-related health issues.

CHAPTER FOURTEEN

An Anglophile Extraordinaire

Between mouthfuls of the main course Dr Dutta would bite into the chilli with gusto, breaking off one small piece at a time until all that was left was the stem. This was a routine that he followed religiously and unfailingly for the two or more years that I spent in South Shields. However to Dr Dutta's credit I must admit he was very generous with his chillies. He passed the bag around the table offering his chillies to anyone brave enough to emulate his habit. There were usually few takers for his offer.

Dr Dutta was the embodiment of the transplanted Indian: a man adrift with no moorings, neither here nor there but wanting to belong somewhere. It appeared that he wanted to obliterate his Indian past and embrace his English present with a finality that would leave no scope for doubt. But try as he did, his Indianness stuck to him like a leech revealing itself in unguarded moments through spontaneous remarks and involuntary quirks that were quintessentially Indian in nature.

The general medicine department in South Shields comprised three separate units – and possibly a fourth if you included the geriatrics branch. Geriatrics and two of the three main units were based at South Shields General while the remaining unit was housed at the Ingham infirmary.

Ingham Infirmary was a much smaller hospital than South Shields General consisting of 180 beds and located a mile down the road from South Shields. The two hospitals, Ingham Infirmary and South Shields General, were administered by a common Health Authority and complemented each other with regard to medical services. South Shields General did not have an accident and emergency department. All emergency admissions were routed through the accident and emergency unit at Ingham.

Each of the three main units had its own special niche of interest: while our unit treated mainly pulmonary or diseases of the lungs, the other unit at South Shields had a particular interest in gastroenterology or diseases of the digestive system. The unit at Ingham specialized in cardiac diseases.

Dr Dutta headed the gastroenterology unit at South Shields and was by far the most interesting personality on the South Shields faculty. He was also the designated clinical educator of the hospital, this status elevating him in the eyes of the house staff and becoming evident in the demeanor he adopted.

We, the recently arrived junior doctors from India, were his guinea pigs, practice targets for the cultural transformation that he was effecting. He directed crude anti-India barbs at us in a show of exaggerated Britishness. Those jabs did hurt, not because they were partly true – like India's abject poverty at that time which we could not deny and accepted – but because of our vulnerability in a foreign land that made it difficult for us to come up with forceful rejoinders.

Dr Dutta would pose a standard question to every new Indian junior doctor who came to South Shields General: Why do you people (Indians) come here (England)?

The psychology behind this question was hard to ascertain. One wondered whether it was genuine concern coming from a senior Indian doctor who had experienced the travails of Britain, or the selfishness of an established immigrant who did not wish his position to be jeopardized by the arrival of more immigrants. Or was it plain embarrassment, the idea of even remotely being associated with these partially unwelcome hillbilly Indian doctors who kept coming to Britain in droves? Anyway, it was not a pleasant question to face and was mostly met with awkward silence.

Dr Dutta was a Bengali. Bengalis are by far the most cerebral of all Indians and there is a common saying that what Bengal thinks today, India thinks tomorrow. It would not be wrong to call Bengal the intellectual laboratory of India. Bengal has been the germinal center for important Indian movements such as the freedom struggle, the Hindu Renaissance and the Communist movement.

During colonial times and in its immediate aftermath Bengal paradoxically also boasted of more than its share of Anglophiles. Anglophilism was almost a religion among the Hindu landed gentry of Bengal in the early 1900s.The extent of this adulation can be gauged by this egregiously exaggerated dedication which appeared in the book, *The Autobiography of an Unknown Indian*written by Nirad Chaudhuri and which stands out as an epitome of Indian servility to Britain.

To the memory of The British Empire in India, which conferred subjecthood on us but withheld citizenship; to which yet every one of us threw out the challenge: "civis britannicus sum," (I am a British Citizen) because all that was good and living within us was made, shaped and quickened by the same British rule.

Nirad Chaudhuri (1897-1999) was a renowned English writer and a self-proclaimed Anglophile extraordinaire of Bengali origin whose prose and incisive writings earned him acclaim abroad and disdain at home. The above-mentioned dedication provoked the wrath of the Indian government with which he was then employed, leading to his termination and loss of pension. Nirad Chaudhuri went on to write more books including *The Continent of Circe*and *Thy Hand Great Anarch*, but he is best remembered for *The Autobiography of an Unknown Indian*and its controversial dedication.

Chaudhuri was a typical Bengali *bhadralok*. *Bhadralok*in Bengali literally means "respectable people" and refers to a privileged class of Bengalis consisting mainly of upper-caste Hindus created by the British during colonial times to assist in ruling the country. For the Bengali *bhadralok*England was the moon and it was almost considered a badge of honor to be educated in England or to be associated with it. Nirad Chaudhuri himself moved to Britain at the ripe old age of 73 where he lived till his death at the age of 101.

Later in life he claimed that the dedication had been misunderstood but the overall thrust of his writings as well as his refutation which stated that "wretched, idiotic, uneducated Indians" had misread his famous lines did little to clarify his stand or assuage the anger felt towards him.

Dr Dutta, like Chaudhuri, was clearly a *bhadralok*or one who had grown up in those traditions. Like many of his compatriots, Dr Dutta had landed on the shores of England in the mid-50s straight out of internship from Calcutta Medical College. That this journey involved a three-month sojourn aboard a cargo ship, which meant inhabiting a musty, cramped room tucked away near the boiler room, was no big deal. It was the price one had to pay to reach the "Promised Land."

In England Dr Dutta had cleared the exams conducted by the Royal College of Physicians with ease. He had then gone one step higher than most run-of-the-mill physicians by obtaining a doctorate from Oxford University. And somewhere along the way to complete his transformation to a "brown saheb" he had acquired a British wife.

Now in his late 50s he attempted to present the picture of an Englishman in all aspects notwithstanding the obvious color of his skin which was immutable. He was a short balding man with residual strands of graying hair that he used to cover his bare pate. Adding pseudo-sophistication to his rounded face was a pointed goatee. Dr Dutta always wore a bow tie instead of a regular tie to set himself apart from the rest. He spoke in a thick, husky voice, made an attempt to pronounce his words carefully and peppered his vocabulary with words that most people would find hard to understand: a clear attempt to demonstrate his erudition.

Funnily enough, his elitist attitude seemed to come apart at the dining table in the cafeteria where we often met for lunch. His palate which had been nurtured on an

Indian diet flavored generously with green chillies seemed to rebel at his attempts to transform himself into a "pucca" Englishmen. Try as hard as he did he could not bring himself to relish the bland English food or overcome his liking for spicy food. To overcome this failing Dr Dutta had a panacea: he carried a small plastic bag containing green chillies wherever he went.

It was a common sight to see Dr Dutta pull out this bag full of chillies from his coat pocket prior to the beginning of every meal. Carefully he would pick out a long green chilli and lay it on the plate beside the food that he was about to imbibe.

Between mouthfuls of the main course Dr Dutta would bite into the chilli with gusto, breaking off one small piece at a time until all that was left was the stem. This was a routine that he followed religiously and unfailingly for the two or more years that I spent in South Shields. However to Dr Dutta's credit I must admit he was very generous with his chilies. He passed the bag around the table offering his chilies to anyone brave enough to emulate his habit. There were usually few takers for his offer.

Dr Dutta never let go of an opportunity to be critical of India or Indian mannerisms. He was adept at searching out obscure aspects of Indian culture for pointed criticism. One evening after we had communicated the demise of a parent to his son, who had received this news with nothing more than a dignified thank you and protracted silence, Dr Dutta launched into a searing commentary on the expression of grief in Indian society. He disdainfully questioned the need for the open expression of grief that accompanied death in Indian society. It was a sign of backwardness, a primitive form of human expression, he pontificated. Compare this dramatic exposition of sorrow with the dignified, sophisticated British attitude, a true mark of a refined culture. Whether one form of expression was superior to the other was a debatable matter and something I was not willing to accept. Nevertheless I found it prudent to remain silent.

CHAPTER FIFTEEN

Britain in Flames

"The whites have become black. A particular sort of violent destructive, nihilistic gangster culture has become the fashion and black and white boys and girls operate in this language together. This language which is wholly false, which is this Jamaican patois that has been intruded in England and that is why so many of us have this sense of literally of a foreign country."

The scenes splashed across the television screen were gory: scowling black youth hurling bricks and bottles at the police, overturning parked vehicles and setting fire to everything in sight.

I had been in South Shields for barely two weeks when race riots broke out, first in Brixton and then throughout the country. I was used to communal riots between Hindus and Muslims in India, but to encounter similar social upheavals in a comparatively advanced country seemed surreal and paradoxical.

Engrossed as I was in overcoming day to day challenges, I'd had little time or reason to look beyond the four walls of the NHS hospitals that had become home to me. The sparse hospital accommodation that I inhabited, the nurses and physicians that I interacted with and the hospital cafeteria that I frequented morning and evening constituted my entire universe. It was as if only the names of towns and cities changed while these basic elements of my daily life remained the same.

Even when I had some spare time I rarely ventured beyond the confines of the hospital establishment. Therefore it was not surprising that I was oblivious to the increasing social unrest that Britain was experiencing and which reached a crescendo in the summer of 1981 in the form of race riots.

By and large these disturbances were not inter-racial riots in the strictest terms. For the greater part public ire was directed toward the police for their high-handed behavior which appeared to have a racial slant. Most of the rioting occurred in predominantly black and Asian areas, but there were instances when one saw groups of black, white and Asian youth jointly battling the police as well.

It would however be inaccurate to completely deny any inter-racial animosity. There were incidents in which white supremacist groups directly clashed with bands of black and Asian youth, and in a suburb of Birmingham black and Asian kids came to loggerheads.

While the epithet "Asian" in Britain is a broad term used to refer to people from the entire subcontinent, the Asian youth involved in these spats were usually of Pakistani and Bangladeshi descent. Indians by and large belonged to a higher socio-economic stratum and desisted from violent conflict prompting even Margaret Thatcher to remark that Indian youth should serve as role models for all Asian youth to emulate. In recent times Indians in Britain prefer to be called British Indians rather than British Asians to avoid being clubbed with Pakistanis and Bangladeshis.

In the months before the riots, the stage was inadvertently being set for this explosion of violence to occur. One of the precipitating factors was the change in police attitude attributed wrongly or rightly to the stern policies of the newly elected government of Margaret Thatcher. To bring the growing crime rate under control the Conservative government vested the police with wide-ranging powers, the most notorious of which was the "Sus laws." Under the "Sus law" the police had the right to stop and search people merely on the basis of suspicion.

Predictably, unemployed black youth in inner city ghettoes became the prime target of this decree. In Asian-dominated areas Asian youth too came under the scanner as the police had the right to question people about their immigrant status under stricter laws. Compounding this unease was the rising unemployment. Unemployment in Britain had skyrocketed from 1.5 million the previous year to a staggering 2.5 million with the colored population accounting for a disproportionately large number.

Sullying the climate even further was Enoch Powell, the inveterate xenophobe who kept harping on the dangers of a "racial civil war." This was the setting in which the riots occurred: first in Brixton and, by mid-summer, the whole of Britain.

Brixton lies in south London and is home to a large West Indian black community which accounts for nearly one-fourth of the population; other immigrant groups are also found residing here in significant numbers. In the summer of 1981 Brixton, along with the rest of Britain, was experiencing the woes of the economic downturn but to an astronomically greater degree. The unemployment rate was twice that of the national average, housing was in short supply, and crime rates were skyrocketing: in other words Brixton was on a short fuse.

Adding to the discomfiture of the local population was the high-handed behavior of the police. In order to curb the growing crime in the area, in early April the Metropolitan police launched Operation Swamp 81, an initiative that deployed hundreds of plain clothes policemen throughout Brixton to implement the Sus law. Close to 1,000 people, mainly black young men, became victims of Operation Swamp 81, fueling a sense of anger in the economically deprived community.

Details of the immediate trigger for the riots that broke out on April 11, 1981 are murky: alleged ill-treatment of an injured black youth and the decision of the police to persist with Operation Swamp 81 despite the mounting anger appear to have been contributing factors.

It was violence on a scale that Britain had never seen before. Starting at 5 p.m. on April 11, 1981, hundreds of black youth (some put the figure close to 5,000) indulged in an orgy of destruction and police defiance using a medley of weapons that included bricks, bottles and petrol bombs. It took nearly 2,500 police personnel to bring the situation under control by 1 a.m. the following day. By then the tally of injured had crossed 300: 299 police personnel and 65 civilians. Over a hundred vehicles including 56 police vehicles had been torched and scores of buildings had been damaged. It was a devastating experience, the first serious riot that Britain had seen in the twentieth century.

After the Brixton riots things subsided and the country experienced relative calm. Except for a few minor incidents of hooliganism everything remained quiet and Britain appeared to be returning to normalcy. However that was not to be.

There was a resurgence of rioting in early July. On July 3, Southall, a western suburb of London that houses the largest concentration of South Asians outside of the subcontinent exploded in anger when a group of Nazi-inspired skinheads beat up an Asian woman en route to a gathering in a local pub. Asian youth retaliated with force and the police had to intervene to protect the skinheads. In the melee the pub was burnt to the ground.

This incident set off a week of rioting that spread from one town to another. Toxeth in Liverpool was the next to follow. The rioting began on the same night as in Southall, when police mistakenly picked up the wrong youth in the case of a stolen motorbike. Here it was a fight between black youth and the police. The black youth used petrol bombs and stones while the police, for the first time in mainland Britain, resorted to the use of CS gas or tear gas in mob control.

What had started off as a battle between blacks and the police soon dragged in white participants and everyone black and white indulged in large-scale looting, a notable feature of these riots. The rioting lasted a total of nine days and was by far the largest of these police–youth confrontations: over 400 police officers were injured, 500 people were arrested and 70 buildings were damaged.

Next in line was Moss Side in Manchester where an unruly mob of over a thousand youth besieged a local police station and injured a policeman. Here, the rioting lasted three days.

Other areas which were the site of major rioting included Chapeltown in Leeds and Handsworth in Birmingham. In Handsworth it was a clash between Asians and blacks. Disturbances of a lesser degree were reported from a host of other towns, from Southhampton in the south to Edinburgh in the north, including Leicester, Sheffield, Portsmouth, Preston, Newcastle, Derby, Nottingham, High Wycombe, Bedford, Wolverhampton, Stockport, Blackburn, Huddersfield, Reading, Chester, and Aldershot. Truly, Britain was in flames. Enoch Powell's premonition of "Rivers of Blood" appeared to be coming true.

Racially charged hate crimes also increased during this period. An especially horrific incident saw five members of an Asian family in Walthamstow (a suburb of London) being killed in an arson attack.

On a personal level, I was fortunate enough not to be caught up in any of the rioting. South Shields, where I was at that time, was a sleepy little town that was immune to these racial tensions. However I did have to skirt this issue when I returned from a visit to India smack in the middle of this rioting in mid-July. Exercising caution, I decided to fly from Heathrow to Newcastle on my way back to South Shields instead of braving a journey by train or bus which would entail contact with the public at large.

*****

Race riots continue to occur in Britain at regular intervals. In the summer of 2001 there was a mini-repeat of 1981 with a series of riots in Oldham, Burnley and Bradford, all areas with a high concentration of Asian immigrants from Pakistan and Bangladesh. Unlike 1981 which was mainly a black protest against police atrocities aggravated by the inequitable socio-economic factors, the subsequent riots in 2001 reflected the tension between the white and the Asian community in certain pockets of the country. To be more accurate these riots almost exclusively involved Asians of Pakistani origin.

The worst affected was Bradford in West Yorkshire that has the second-largest concentration of Asians of any UK city. Asians here total close to 100,000 and constitute roughly 20 percent of the population in this ethnically segregated city which has always had a history of troubled relations between the majority white community and the Asian community.

In a round of rioting that lasted two or three days and was partly provoked by fears of an impending march by a whites-only right wing group, nearly 100 youth indulged in uncontrolled looting and arson. More than 300 police officers were injured, 297 arrests were made and 200 jail sentences totaling 604 years were passed out, making it the highest for any riot in Britain.

Riots again engulfed Britain in 2011. As usual the trigger for the rioting was an incident involving the police and members of the black community. This time the site of the altercation was Tottenham in North London: on August 4, a black man, Mark Duggan, a father of four, was killed in an altercation with the police. Two days later a peaceful protest march by members of the black community deteriorated into a free-for-all with masked hoodlums going on a rampage of arson and looting.

The next day the rioting spread to other parts of London like Brixton, a racial tinderbox that has been the venue of several riots over the years and was the focal point of the infamous riots of 1981. Other areas affected included Enfield, Islington and Hackney, all areas with significant black populations. By day 4, rioting had spread to cities outside of London with both Birmingham and Manchester reporting incidents of violence.

What had started off as a running confrontation between blacks and the police took on an inter-communal slant in some instances. Notable among these was a horrific incident in Birmingham in which a car driven by a black rioter ploughed through a group of Asians who had gathered to protect their properties from looters, killing three young Asians in the process.

Commentators pointed to the stern austerity measures imposed by the Cameron government as the real reason for this outbreak of violence. The spree of rioting that had England up in flames in 1981 had also taken place against the backdrop of an economic downturn.

More disconcerning was the general lawlessness that prevailed. A sizable proportion of the masked hoodlums were also whites, indicating that the mayhem had degenerated into a free-for-all that cut across racial lines in which personal gain rather than social protest had become the primary motto.

But the collective British persona is not willing to accept the ugliness of riots that have come to be a part of British life. Neither is it willing to acknowledge the fact that whites too have become a part of the decadence. British racism and immigrant phobia, never far below the surface, found vent through remarks such as this.

David Starkey, a well-known historian and TV personality commented on BBC:

> "*The whites have become black. A particular sort of violent destructive, nihilistic gangster culture has become the fashion and black and white boys and*

girls operate in this language together. This language which is wholly false, which is this Jamaican patois that has been intruded in England and that is why so many of us have this sense of literally of a foreign country."

CHAPTER SIXTEEN

A Royal Wedding

But this scene reminded me of the Middle Ages when servile masses would erupt in joy at royal events such as weddings and coronations, events designed to distract the common peasants from the drudgery of their banal lives. Shorn of their colonial empire that had disintegrated by the 1960s, the British seemingly needed this prop of royalty to give them a sense of identity, to lift up their sagging morale in a fast-changing world that had reduced them from a colonial superpower to just another player.

The proclamation had all the mien of a medieval kingdom. Only the external trappings were different. The frocked herald with his over-sized trumpet and the drummer boys were missing. Instead, the Lord Chancellor, a senior ranking member of the government, dressed in modern clothes made the announcement via television. He gushed obsequiously: "It is with greatest pleasure that the Queen and the Duke of Edinburgh announce the betrothal of their beloved son the Prince of Wales to the Lady Diana Spencer, daughter of the Earl Spencer and the Honorable Mrs. Shand Kydd."

Not to be outdone, Prime Minister Margaret Thatcher joined in the chorus and led members from both Houses of Parliament in expressing “great pleasure”, at this development

Feudal servility was a trait that was quite common in post-independence India, a hangover from colonial times and the age of the maharajas. The disadvantaged exhibited an extraordinary subservience to the elite, and helpless serfs would prostrate themselves in front of landlords. Such behavior can be explained away by the widespread illiteracy, poverty and a colonial mindset that the British had forced upon the people of India.

But to see similar behavior among a majority of Brits was something of a surprise. I had expected a more refined and enlightened conduct in one of the foremost countries of the world which boasted of a literacy rate greater than 90 percent and which had led the world in implementing parliamentary democracy.

That a personal matter like an engagement should be treated as an event of national concern was something that I could not comprehend. I scoured my memory for a comparable event in India but found none. Yes, we had our own political dynasty in India, the Nehru-Gandhi clan which had to some extent replaced the maharajas of the past. And yes, weddings in India were celebrated with pomp and glory. Nonetheless, even the weddings of the progeny of the rich and powerful never assumed the degree of national importance that I was witnessing in Britain.

An unabashed exhibition of servility was in full display in the months leading up to the wedding with the press playing a central role. The media frenzy began in February when the engagement of Charles and Diana was officially announced: the date was February 24, 1981.

Since then, not a day passed without a picture of the couple appearing prominently in one newspaper or the other. An incident that created some controversy comes to mind: it involved a photo that appeared in the media soon after the engagement was announced. Diana was working as a nursery teacher in a London school at the time and the picture showed Diana with two small children, one astride her hips and the other holding her hand. Diana herself came through as a rare combination of beauty and shyness. What provoked the controversy however was the contour of her legs that was highlighted by the sunlight shining through her sheer skirt. Diana reportedly cried after seeing those pictures.

Tabloids were agog with every new detail of this royal romance and major newspapers appeared keen not to be left behind. Diana's engagement ring was another hot topic that evoked intense scrutiny. Newspapers described how Diana deviated from tradition and picked out a ring from the Garrard Jeweler's catalog, rather than have one custom-made. Garrard Jewelers is a jewelry firm that has served the British monarchy for over a hundred years and is in charge of maintenance and supervision of the royal jewelry.

Every minute aspect of the ring was covered in great detail in newspaper columns. The cost, they told us, was 30,000 pounds. Some reporters waxed eloquent about the type of gold that was used and argued extensively about the origin of the yellow metal in question, whether it was from Welsh gold mines in keeping with the tradition of

British royalty. Others chose to comment at length on the 14 diamonds surrounding the central sapphire detailing their carat value and history. And all described in exquisite detail the oval blue sapphire that formed the central piece of the ring.

The royal wedding of Charles and Diana took place in the July of 1981 and offered a welcome respite to the country after a torrid summer of race riots. To me this event provided another insight into the British mind. The pomp and pageantry on the D-Day was impressive. It was a resplendent affair worth watching. Princess Diana looked beautiful in a gorgeous ivory taffeta wedding gown that reportedly cost 9,000 pounds and sported a 25-foot train. Prince Charles was clad in the uniform of a naval commander and looked handsome. But it was quite obvious even then that it was Princess Diana who was the star of the show. Prince Charles was 32 and Lady Diana was 20 years of age.

A national holiday had been declared and it appeared that all of Britain was glued to its seats that day watching the proceedings on TV. Each and every TV channel carried the event live. Worldwide a total of 750 million people watched the wedding and that included 55 million Americans who woke up early in the morning before 6 a.m. to view this royal wedding.

Nearly 600,000 people lined the streets to watch Diana and Charles en route to St Paul's Cathedral, the site of the wedding. The guest list at the actual wedding ceremony numbered around 3,500 and included presidents, prime ministers, kings and queens from 58 countries.

The ceremony itself was notable in that Lady Diana chose to omit the word "obey" from the wedding vows in keeping with modern times. There were a couple of glitches: Diana muddled up Charles's full name calling him "Philip Charles..." rather than "Charles, Philip...." Charles too fumbled with the wording of his vows.

The crowd worked itself into a mad frenzy when the newlyweds emerged on the balcony of Buckingham Palace and gave the audience what it had been waiting for: the post-nuptial kiss that was one long, lingering moment carrying the crowds outside to the heights of ecstasy.

But this scene reminded me of the Middle Ages when servile masses would erupt in joy at royal events such as weddings and coronations, events designed to distract the common peasants from the drudgery of their banal lives. Shorn of their colonial empire that had disintegrated by the 1960s, the British seemingly needed this prop of royalty to give them a sense of identity, to lift up their sagging morale in a fast-changing world that had reduced them from a colonial superpower to just another player.

India on the other hand and had moved far ahead, adopting an egalitarian approach by relegating its maharajas and maharanis to the status of ordinary citizens in keeping with the principles of modern times. The 26th amendment to the Constitution of India passed in 1971 virtually stripped all former princely rulers of both their titles and the monetary sustenance they had been receiving from the government (Privy Purses) since independence.

The British Empire in India had consisted of two broad administrative categories: British India, which included territories under the direct control of Britain, and princely states, which consisted of native kingdoms whose rulers had ceded authority to the British through treaties and had been allowed to remain as nominal rulers. These rulers carried exalted titles like "Maharajah" and "Nizam" but were mere puppets who worked under the supervision of locally-placed British political officers or "Agents."

Incensed with the idea of having to vacate India, Britain had thrown a monkey wrench into the transition by giving these princely rulers the choice to join either India or Pakistan or to remain as separate kingdoms, which was bound to create more chaos in an already uncertain and fractious environment. In order to harmoniously incorporate these territories into India, India's new rulers negotiated a deal with these princes that guaranteed them an annual payment, a Privy Purse commensurate with the size of their kingdoms, and allowed them to retain their honorifics. But 25 years later, India thought it appropriate to discard this vestige of feudality and scrapped this entitlement.

CHAPTER SEVENTEEN

A Depressing Failure

And I paid the price for my stubbornness: I failed again. According to the official classification, it was a "bare failure" (as opposed to a "clear failure" or a "bad failure") which meant that I had just fallen short of the passing mark. Nevertheless, it was a failure and my morale hit rock bottom. Self-doubt resurfaced with a vengeance. I wondered whether I had it in me to succeed. Was it all a mistake? Maybe I should have never left India. Was it perhaps time to call it quits and return to India?

"One day, you too must become like him," my mother had turned to me and said as I stood on the platform of the Cantonment Railway station in Bangalore tightly clutching her hand. I was barely 5 years old. She was referring to my granduncle standing by the side of the *Island Express*train which he was about to board. The year was 1959 and he was on his way to Cochin to make the long sea journey to England- to study for the FRCS.

My mother had grown up in a small hamlet of not more than 20 dwellings in southern India along the current Karnataka- Maharashtra border and had barely managed to matriculate from high school after her parents moved to a bigger town. But the importance of education was not lost on her; a gritty ambitious woman whose intrinsic drive and vision far surpassed her educational qualifications, she was bent on ensuring that her two sons attained the highest educational level possible which perforce included a stint abroad. Uncles and cousins who had done well were constantly being held up as models for us to emulate. It was through her that I first heard about these English qualifications: MRCP and FRCS.

These suffixes evoked a great deal of admiration during my growing up years in India. At that time I was unaware of what they stood for. Not many adults seemed to know what the letters meant. Nevertheless everyone seemed impressed by their mere mention. It signified a higher degree of learning; it set that particular physician apart from the rest of the crowd and defined him/her as a superior professional.

MRCP stands for "Member of the Royal College of Physicians" and FRCS is the abbreviation for "Fellow of the Royal College of Surgeons." Though they were both postgraduate degrees, the British qualifications carried more weightage in the Indian mind than local Indian postgraduate degrees which required a structured learning that spanned three years, were more rigorous and involved the writing of a research thesis.

The Royal Colleges initially began as licensing bodies for physicians and surgeons. There are three main colleges located in the UK: London, Edinburgh, and Glasgow. The Royal College based in Dublin, Ireland is considered a sister institution. The Royal College of Physicians, London was the first to be created in 1518 following a royal charter by King Henry the VIII. Glasgow and Edinburgh got their own Royal Colleges in 1599 and 1681 respectively. The Royal College of Physicians, Ireland was founded in 1654.

The Royal College of Surgeons, distinct from the Royal College of Physicians, has a more interesting origin. Surgery as a specialty traces its roots to the trade of barbering. In fact the first surgeons were barbers and were called barber-surgeons performing tonsorial operations along with limited surgical procedures that were in vogue at that time like bloodletting. Over time however, the barber–surgeons acquired a distinct identity of their own and came to be known as surgeons.

The primary intent of these bodies, when founded, was to oversee the practice of medicine which till then had no regulating body. These fraternities were involved in issuing licenses and censuring malpractice. Today these Royal Colleges are known throughout the realm of the ex-British Empire more for the certifying exams that they conduct.

The exam itself consists of two parts. Part I is exclusively a written exam consisting of multiple-choice questions. In my time there were 60 main questions with 5 sub-questions, each to be marked “True” or “False.” Not only did the limited number of questions fail to do justice to the extensive syllabus involved but the process of negative marking made the exam more onerous as well. Negative marking meant that you lost 1 point for every wrong answer. Therefore it was prudent to leave a question unanswered to save yourself the loss of a point in situations of uncertainty. The presence of negative marking led to complex strategizing with candidates hotly debating amongst themselves as to how many questions had to be attempted and how many to be left blank to ensure the best chance of success. Fortunately in recent times the MRCP (UK) Board has done away with negative marking.

In addition to a written component Part 2 had a clinical exam that brought you face-to-face with actual patients and human examiners and added a degree of subjectivity to the process of failing and passing.

For a foreign physician pursuing a career in the UK, passing the MRCP or FRCS exams is a required rite of passage, a stamp that indicates that you have "arrived" and are on par with UK trained physicians. At the outset these exams appear as a routine professional certifying procedure, but in reality each is a complex ordeal invariably punctuated by repeated failures and one that demands not only knowledge of the subject but also the grit to overcome what was seen by many foreign physicians as discriminatory practices in the conduct of these exams.

It was common knowledge that foreign physicians were subject to a more rigorous scrutiny than the locals, something that was never officially acknowledged but openly admitted to in day-to-day conversations by native English consultants. The explanation most often offered for these double standards was that countries like India, Bangladesh, Nigeria and Uganda do not have strict regulatory systems in place and it was the bounden duty of the British to make sure that untrained physicians were not let loose on the people.

A study sanctioned by the MRCP Board in 2010 confirmed what foreign physicians had always suspected: lower pass rates when compared to local graduates. While local graduates had pass rates ranging between 60 and 70 percent for Part 1, international or foreign graduates registered rates between 40 and 50 percent. These differences were even more marked in the clinical part : 70-80 percent for UK graduates and 40 to 60 percent for foreign graduates.

A sub-analysis of the data proved to be even more of an eye-opener. If you were white your chances of passing were better in either category: white UK graduates and white foreign graduates fared better than their colored counterparts. Even if most of these differences can be attributed to the disparate medical school backgrounds of the candidates as claimed by the study authors, this factor alone does not explain the entire picture. Why does a white UK graduate fare better than a non-white UK graduate? There is undeniably an element of racism even in professional British circles.

I plunged into the MRCP process as soon as I could. Within three months of landing in the UK I had appeared for Part I. The result that came six weeks later was disappointing to say the least: I had failed; the first failure in my academic career. Having had a stellar academic record and graduated from one of the top medical schools in India, it was difficult for me to stomach this setback. Compounding my failure was the alien environment: a distant unfriendly country. I felt miserable.

After wallowing in self-pity for a few days I pulled myself together and decided to take another crack at the exam without any respite. I had reached South Shields in March of 1981 and the next exam was slated for May. I decided to go for it ignoring the sage advice of my friends who had suggested that the September date would be more appropriate as it would give me a full six months to prepare.

And I paid the price for my stubbornness: I failed again. According to the official classification, it was a "bare failure" (as opposed to a "clear failure" or a "bad failure") which meant that I had just fallen short of the passing mark. Nevertheless, it was a failure and my morale hit rock bottom. Self-doubt resurfaced with a vengeance. I wondered whether I had it in me to succeed. Was it all a mistake? Maybe I should have never left India. Was it perhaps time to call it quits and return to India?

During these dark moments I had frightening visions of my quest ending right here in the UK. I envisioned myself sometime in the future wandering aimlessly and hopelessly through gloomy geriatric wards.

After another protracted bout of self-pity I gathered myself and attempted to chart out a strategy to pull myself out of the quagmire of repeated failures. There must be a way out of all this, I told myself. Why not take the MRCP (I) exam which was conducted by the Royal College of Physicians of Dublin? Part 1 of the exam consisted of exactly the same question paper as that of MRCP (UK), only that it was conducted under the aegis of the Royal College of Physicians of Dublin. I had also heard that the pass rate was higher with the marking being more lenient.

Thus, in the fall of 1981 I traveled to Dublin, wrote the exam and passed at the first attempt. It was a great relief. But that success committed me to going back to Dublin for Part 2: it was a minor hurdle and I could live with that.

CHAPTER EIGHTEEN

A Low Blow

And when I went to Carol for the umpteenth time to make sure that my reference letters had been dispatched in a timely manner, she sensed the consternation in my mind and took pity on me. After furtively looking around, she motioned me to sit down in front of her, pulled out a copy of Dr Peter's reference letter and pointed to its conclusion.

Sarah Peters was her name. She was young - probably in her mid-thirties with cascading blond hair and light blue eyes, quite the opposite of the typical consultant – a 40 to 50 year old dowdy-looking male. But when she spoke, a cynical smirk appeared on her face, making one a trifle uncomfortable- a hint that beneath the pleasant exterior was another person and a signal that one had to be on guard.

The four and a half months that we spent under the tutelage of Dr Anthony was a placid period that did not call for major behavioral adjustments. But that phase was soon to be over. Dr Anthony was a locum and his tenure was coming to an end. He was to be replaced by Dr.Peters, a local UK graduate who was just finishing up her senior registrar training in Newcastle. We had already heard a great deal about her from Dr Dutta who just couldn't stop extolling her virtues; he went on and on about how accomplished and how smart she was.

My colleague and I had been retained for the regular SHO positions. That was a relief. But a new consultant meant we had to start all over again: a new period of adjustment loomed before us. We had to adapt ourselves to the new consultant's work pattern and tailor our style of working to suit her likes and dislikes. We had become pretty comfortable working under Dr Anthony and did not look forward to this change. Nevertheless we had no choice and braced ourselves for the challenge.

Dr Peters was a trained gastroenterologist, but after waiting unsuccessfully for several years for an opening to turn up in her field of interest, she had opted to accept this position as a consultant in chest medicine. I could not help but notice the element of discrimination in her appointment. Dr Anthony had the necessary qualifications required for a chest physician; yet he was making way for another consultant who lacked the requisite expertise: the foreigner element was undoubtedly the tipping factor.

The fact that Dr Peters was not a trained chest physician was obvious when she took charge. She was hesitant in dealing with lung disorders and became excessively defensive when my colleague and I asked her routine harmless questions. Our intention was not to put her on the spot. We were merely attempting to assuage our medical curiosity. But she usually reacted to our queries with a piqued retort and that put an end to our case discussions on rounds.

Though the period of adjustment could not be termed as overtly hostile it was not a smooth ride either. My colleague, who was at least five years older than I, and who had worked for a couple of years as a consultant in New Delhi before coming to the UK, handled the situation much better. His post-medical school experience made him more mature in understanding the day-to-day professional conflicts that physicians face and he was able to soon establish a good rapport with Dr Peters.

In contrast, my relationship with Dr Peters took on a rocky course. There were issues on either side that contributed to a sense of uneasiness in our interaction. Looking back, I realize that I was not the easiest of subordinates to work with. I was cocky and even a trifle arrogant, an attitude I had unconsciously imbibed as a result of being educated in an elite institution and which was rooted in the false impression that I was intellectually superior to my colleagues. Added to this negative attribute was the serious loss of confidence that I had suffered in my early days in the UK as a result of exam failures and the inability to land a job of my liking. I attempted to compensate for my setbacks with an overt display of my medical knowledge. To put it bluntly, I had an unfortunate tendency to show off.

Dr Peters was a new consultant, a position that says you have arrived, but which also invests you with a responsibility and an independence that can be scary. As a consultant you have no one to turn to. There is no one looking over your shoulder. You are it. Your decisions, right or wrong, are yours. And having a smart aleck junior questioning every decision of yours it is not the best of situations. I can relate to her reaction better now after working as a consultant myself.

Though we fell into a routine and carried on with our work, we were never able to fully overcome or forget the initial reservations that we had about each other. They lingered on and were to resurface with negative consequences for me when I finished my tenure on the unit one and a half years later.

Towards the end of my term in South Shields, I began looking for a registrar position. I had worked for 18 months as a senior house officer and I felt that I was ready to move up in the hierarchy to the level of a registrar. To land a registrar job with the amount of experience that I had was a reasonable expectation. Nonetheless, all my efforts met with little success.

There appeared to be a glitch somewhere. My résumé was quite impressive and I featured on the shortlist on many occasions. However it was at the final stage which involved a face-to-face interview and a review of one's reference letters that I was found wanting.

After returning from six interviews empty-handed, I began to wonder about the reasons for my failure. Was it my personality? Was it my ethnicity? Or was it something more mundane like an adverse recommendation letter?

Dr Peters, by virtue of being my latest boss, was one of my referees. I had assumed that after working with her for over a year she would have forgiven me for my initial intemperate behavior. But that wasn't the case.

I found this out accidentally and I must thank Carol, Dr Peter's secretary, for that. Carol was a warm personable young lady with whom I had developed a professional but friendly rapport during my stay in South Shields. And when I went to Carol for the umpteenth time to make sure that my reference letters had been dispatched in a timely manner, she sensed the consternation in my mind and took pity on me. After furtively looking around she motioned me to sit down in front of her, pulled out a copy of Dr Peter's reference letter and pointed to its conclusion.

For the most part it was a stereotyped recommendation letter that followed the usual format but at the end Dr Peters had, it appeared deliberately, thrown in a phrase to queer the pitch: "at times he is unsure of himself."

A few words like these in a recommendation letter are sufficient to quash one's chances of success. So, for my next job application, I switched referees putting down the name of a consultant from a previous job. Lo and behold, I landed the job easily.

Looking back at this incident with an objective eye nearly 30 years later, I can say that Dr Peters may not have been completely off the mark. But it was a subtle attempt at sabotage, a nuanced remark intentionally left open to interpretation that was most likely to be negative and one that lacked an in-depth analysis of my hesitancy. In short, it was a statement that could have well been avoided but wasn't for ulterior reasons.

I am a cautious physician by disposition, extremely cognizant of the fact that my decision can tilt the scales between life and death. Even later in my career, I would be accused of not being "aggressive." But to me "aggression" is not a word that one should use in the practice of medicine: it has the connotation of bulldozing one's way through.

Many physicians are under the impression that they are obligated to do something regardless of whether it is right or wrong when a patient presents himself or herself to them. Such an attitude often results in unnecessary tests and rash decisions that can lead to adverse outcomes.

*Primum non nocere*is a Latin phrase that means "First, do no harm" and it is a cardinal precept that is ingrained in all medical students. To this day I strongly subscribe to this adage, pausing and thinking twice before embarking on any decision related to the medical care of a patient. The human body is a resilient and wondrous organ with an infinite capacity to rejuvenate and take care of itself. The most important thing for a physician to know is when to intervene and when not to. And many a time, a decision to not do anything is in the best interest of the patient.

CHAPTER NINETEEN

PLAY AT WORK

One afternoon when the fire alarm went off, amidst the clanging of bells, the sirens from fire engines and the hustle and bustle of occupants rushing out of the building, we found an embarrassed Krishnakumar trying to sneak out of the back door with his girlfriend, both of them clad in nothing more than a bath towel.

One thing was certain. The UK – or rather the NHS in the 1980s – was not prudish. Flirting was common between nurses and doctors. It was not unusual to find dainty nurses clad in short skirts perched playfully on the consultant's lap especially during the festivities associated with Christmas and New Year's Day. Nobody thought too much about this.

Indian physicians and British nurses in particular enjoyed a unique chemistry, an affinity that transcended ethnicity and national differences and one that was not colored by acrimonious historical events. It was a relationship driven by the inherent natural attraction between the sexes. During my initial locum phase I had little time to appreciate these interesting friendly interactions as each stay was too short to get to know people. It was in South Shields that I had the luxury of understanding these dalliances and observe these relationships from close quarters, especially through the romps of my fellow junior physicians.

When I look back at this chapter of my stay in the UK, the first person who comes to my mind is Roberts. Roberts was a fellow SHO who hailed from the southern Indian state of Kerala. He was a good five years older than I and had spent several years navigating his way through Gulf countries before landing in the UK. The word "experienced" was what one would use to describe Roberts's skill with women; he had a way with them. He was the "love guru" of our small band of young physicians from south Asia, one who routinely gave homilies of succeeding with the opposite sex and was ever eager to give tips to those of us in need of expert advice. Nurses adored him not only because of his stocky physique but also for the sweet words that emanated from his mouth. He was the essence of friendliness; he was always seen with a disarming smile on his mustachioed face.

During weekends it was difficult to catch a glimpse of Roberts as he kept himself "busy". A "Do not disturb" sign hung on his door knob made it clear that he had no time for us.

Roberts' first and only rule for success was: *be nice*. If one was nice, he would pontificate, physical attributes became secondary. He was convinced that girls prefer a "nice person" to "a good looker on an ego trip." This adage of his seemed to strike a chord with Krishnakumar.

Krishnakumar was the exact opposite of Roberts. He was not someone that you would describe as handsome by any stretch of imagination. In fact he was the classic example of a simpleton; innocence dripped from his face. He was gawky, embarrassingly scrawny and extremely shy. He found it hard to go through a full sentence in the presence of a woman. A pair of thick glasses adorned his face to complete a picture of diffidence.

He looked at Roberts's exploits with awe and admiration and secretly nursed a desire to emulate him. I found him locked in conversation with Roberts for hours together, trying to garner the intricacies of interaction between the sexes.

A few months down the line I began to see less and less of Krishnakumar. He no longer frequented the doctors' lounge which had been his traditional haunt. On confronting him one day he let out his secret. Roberts had proved to be a successful teacher and he, Krishnakumar, now had a girlfriend.

Krishnakumar soon got carried away by his new-found confidence and began dating two women simultaneously: one was a nurse who worked with him and the other was a young nursing student. He seemed to have become a veteran at handling the opposite sex in just a short span of time. I found it hard at times to comprehend the change that had occurred in him. He even formulated a schedule: entertaining one of his girlfriends in his room at lunchtime between 1 and 2 p.m. while reserving the evening hours for the other. Whether his girlfriends knew of this arrangement, I am not sure. But as South Shields was a small place and this was common knowledge, I presume they must have been aware. Relationships in this setting, in most cases, were purely physical and transient without any emotional baggage, long-term expectations or commitments.

Krishnakumar's afternoon sex sessions did land him in a soup one day. He was literally caught in the act. False fire alarms were a common occurrence in our doctors' complex. One afternoon when the fire alarm went off, amidst the clanging of bells, the sirens from fire engines and the hustle and bustle of occupants rushing out of the building, we found an embarrassed Krishnakumar trying to sneak out of the back door with his girlfriend, both of them clad in nothing more than a bath towel. We had a big laugh at his expense. From then on Krishnakumar made it a point to drop his afternoon rendezvous. He also made the wise decision to stick to one girlfriend.

While the majority of doctor-nurse friendships fostered here were transient affairs, interactions that one would describe as a fling, there were some relationships that went beyond pure fun to assume a serious nature. Suraj's fondness for Kirin fell into the latter category. Suraj was a fellow SHO who worked in the cardiology ward. Kirin too worked in the same unit: she was one of the junior nurses. Suraj and Kirin took a liking for each other from day one. They had personalities that matched. Both were soft-spoken, modest in their behavior and not given to an excessive display of exuberance. They liked indoor activities like cooking, watching TV and chatting with each other. To use the cliché, they were made for each other – or so it seemed.

For almost two years they courted each other. Suraj even confessed to me one day that Kirin was the type of girl that he would like to marry. But there was a problem. Suraj belonged to a high-caste, wealthy Hindu family from Delhi that was extremely conservative in its outlook. His parents would never allow him to proceed with such an alliance and he, the obedient son, just did not have the courage to oppose their views. So one day Suraj resigned his job, went back to Delhi, married the girl of his parents' liking and settled down there. What happened to Kirin I don't know. Probably she too moved on with her life.

But there were other romantic encounters that did have a happy ending. A colleague of mine from a neighboring hospital was besotted with a young student nurse. He married her, moved to the US and had three beautiful children, two girls and a boy. Thirty years later they are still together and madly in love, I am told.

Part Three

Uncertainty Again

CHAPTER TWENTY

HOPE AND DISAPPOINTMENT

For a moment, I wondered whether I was in the US and whether this was New York. Trash was all over the place, on the pavement, in the middle of the street, and in front of doorsteps, mounds of it emanating a foul odor that was suffocating. Crumbling red brick buildings with broken windows and termite-infested doors interspersed with empty unkempt lots teeming with runaway weeds completed the picture of decay. More frightening to me however were the bands of unruly bulky youth with beer cans in their hands idling by the roadside and whose glances in my direction seemed to say, "What is this guy doing here? Looks like he is easy prey."

Written in bold letters across the fifth page of my passport was a clear directive to officials in the US: MAXIMUM STAY THREE WEEKS. EXTENSION NOT RECOMMENDED.

Nevertheless, I was overjoyed. My visa request had been approved and I was free to travel to the United States for a job interview. Several of my colleagues had been felled at this stage with their application for a visa being denied. I had successfully cleared one more hurdle.

Getting to the US is an obstacle race for a foreign physician. Stacked along the way are numerous hurdles of varying difficulty quotients, each requiring a different set of skills to negotiate. The first and easiest of these barriers is the Qualifying Exam (a rigorous test of one's medical knowledge spread out over two full days). I classify this difficult examination as an easy undertaking because the outcome could be crafted to a great extent by one's own efforts.

The second obstacle – obtaining a tourist visa to the US to attend a job interview – was, in contrast, totally dependent on the whims of the consular officer at the American embassy. Getting a tourist visa for a single young Indian male was almost an impossible task in those days. The adjectives listed above were red flags that marked one out as a potential immigrant to the US and someone who was likely to stay back in the US after gaining entry via a tourist visa.

Deportation from the shores of the US is usually a lengthy legal process which the authorities wished to avoid by adopting a preventive approach. It was easier to deny one a tourist visa than to get one deported later. Therefore, potential candidates were carefully scrutinized before being issued a visa and rejected on the slightest suspicion.

The consular authorities required a long list of documents including a return ticket, documented evidence of a permanent job, a copy of a recent bank statement and the most important requirement of all: written proof of one's purpose of traveling to the US. A sightseeing venture was certain to be shot down promptly. I had with me a letter on an official letterhead from Grand Hospital in Chicago inviting me for an interview. Unlike my colleagues who preferred to personally go down to London to apply for a visa, I opted for the mail option and waited expectantly for an answer. Luckily my gamble paid off.

But there were two more obstacles to be tackled. First, I had to obtain a residency position and second, the process of getting legalized in the US with a work permit and a Green Card. These were formidable propositions and even thinking about them made me break out into a cold sweat. I calmed myself by saying that I would cross the Tiber when I came to it.

Lack of advance planning has been a personal quirk that I have found difficult to shake off. Looking back, I am appalled at my sheer stupidity. I landed in New York without a definite place to stay or a modus operandi to land an interview for a residency. Not surprisingly, I ran into problems from the moment I landed in New York.

A friend of my cousin who was supposed to pick me up from the airport and accommodate me in his apartment failed to materialize. Fortunately for me, another friend of my cousin who had landed in New York earlier that day was in the same sorry plight: his contact too had failed to turn up. The two of us got together and decided to check into a Holiday Inn a short distance from the airport.

The hotel was not in the best of locations: the area surrounding it had a rundown deserted look. The streets were empty, shop doors were shuttered, windows were barricaded with sheets of plywood and the infamous New York graffiti was visible all over. The hotel receptionist, a mousy little man with thick glasses and a shock of unkempt red hair, only added to my discomfort by warning me in a conspiratorial tone of the dangers of venturing out into the vicinity: a crime-ridden area where muggings were common. So, for two days, we did not step out of the hotel. Instead my new friend and I spent our time holed up in the hotel making telephone calls, trying desperately to find someone who would give us a place to stay and pleading with brusque hospital secretaries to grant us a job interview.

On day three we finally left the hotel. My friend was able to trace a long-lost college-mate who was kind enough to put him up and I moved to Morristown, New Jersey to stay with an Indian family, distant relatives of my cousin.

The next few days saw me travelling every day from Morristown to New York by bus to look for a job. The commute lasted an hour but was comfortable as the bus was well heated and had spacious seats. Once within the city however I had to transfer to the subway system to find my way about.

The New York subway was quite different from the London Underground: the carriages were dirtier and had graffiti all over them. The seats lacked cushions and the compartments were jam-packed most of the time. Some of the subway stations, especially the ones in Bronx and in Brooklyn, were downright scary even during daytime, with long stretches of dimly-lit isolated platforms with drunks sprawled out on the floor and disheveled vagabonds squatting near the entrance. It was not a pleasant experience to travel by the New York subway although I must admit it was fast and convenient. Additionally, it was inexpensive. You could travel from one end of the subway system to the other for just 75 cents.

My calls to land an interview had yielded some results. Two hospitals, one in Brooklyn and the other in Bronx, had given me interview dates. My first appointment was with Brooklyn Hospital Center. The easiest way to get to the hospital, I was told by the secretary, was by subway, and the closest stop was Dekalb Ave on the B line. The interview being set for 1.30 p.m., I promptly alighted from the train at 12.30 p.m., a good one hour before my scheduled time. When I emerged from the subway station on to the street above, I was a little perplexed. The whole stretch of the road was empty: not a soul was in sight; the scene resembled a ghost town from a Western movie. I hurried down the street to the hospital occasionally glancing over my shoulder to ensure that I wasn't being followed. The interview proved to be uneventful and I never heard back from them.

My interview at the Bronx Lebanon Hospital gave me a little more hope. Getting to the hospital proved to be more complicated than my visit to the Brooklyn Hospital Center: first I had to travel by subway, then transfer to a bus and finally cover the last half mile on foot. As I stepped down from the bus the scene that met my eye was appalling. For a moment I wondered whether I was in the US and whether this was New York. Trash was all over the place, on the pavement, in the middle of the street and in front of doorsteps, mounds of it emanating a foul odor that was suffocating. Crumbling red brick buildings with broken windows and termite-infested doors interspersed with empty unkempt lots teeming with runaway weeds completed the picture of decay. More frightening to me however were the bands of unruly bulky youth with beer cans in their hands idling by the roadside and whose glances in my direction seemed to say, "What is this guy doing here? Looks like he is easy prey." This was south Bronx, one of New York City's impoverished neighborhoods that had a high crime rate.

It would be an understatement if I said I stood out in these surroundings. I was smartly clad in a well-ironed suit, a silk tie and shiny shoes – my interview gear – and was all of 5 feet 4 inches tall. In a physical confrontation, I knew I didn't stand a chance. With my eyes focused on the road ahead and making a conscious effort to ignore these seemingly rowdy elements I walked on. I heaved a sigh of relief when I reached the entrance to the hospital.

The cardiologist who interviewed me was duly impressed by my credentials and promised me that I would be ranked high up on the match-list. This specific hospital had a track record of hiring Indian medical graduates, particularly those who had additional training in the UK, and my interviewer's encouraging assurance gave me a glimmer of hope.

An interview was only the first step of getting into a residency program. The next and more important aspect was the matching program, an elaborate process by which aspiring candidates and hospitals are paired together.

When hospitals were done interviewing their quota of eligible candidates, they would draw up a list in order of their preference. It was a list that was influenced not purely by merit. US graduates were expectedly the first choice regardless of their credentials. For foreign graduates, additional factors like visa status played a significant role in getting on to this list.

Graduates like me who did not have a visa to work in the US needed to be sponsored by a hospital prior to employment. Not all hospitals were eligible to sponsor a candidate: only those located in rural areas with paucity of physicians or inner-city hospitals catering to impoverished sections of society could do so. For a hospital, sponsoring a foreign physician also meant contending with the immigration department whose vagaries could be highly unpredictable and prolonged. No hospital wanted to have a situation in July, when residencies would begin, wherein a physician could not start work because of an unresolved visa issue. Therefore, hospitals were hesitant to match a candidate without a visa: only in the case of exceptional candidates did they do so.

Like hospitals, candidates too were expected to make up a rank list reflecting one's preference. These separate confidential lists (strictly speaking, hospitals are not supposed to indicate to candidates whether they would match them) were then submitted to a central body that matched them together giving candidates the right of first choice as long as the candidate figured anywhere in the particular hospital's match list. The match list was a farce for foreign medical graduates for whom even a single interview was hard to come by.

The results of the matching program are published in March every year. A match opened up the possibility of a career in the US; if not it meant at least one more year of struggle and uncertainty.

I attended one other unpromising interview at a Veterans' Administration hospital in New Jersey and I was not hopeful of landing a position there.

After a busy three weeks in New York, I returned to South Shields and waited nervously for the match results. I was pretty hopeful that I would match with the Bronx-Lebanon hospital. But when the match results came out on March 16, I drew a naught. Half of me wanted to give up and turn back; the other half egged me on. I was once again at a loss.

CHAPTER TWENTY-ONE

A Taste of British Jingoism

The Sun, a tabloid newspaper, assumed a singularly notorious role, arrogating to itself the voice of the country and becoming the official cheerleader for Margaret Thatcher. One headline read: "Stick it up your Junta." On another occasion, when the Royal Navy submarine HMS Conqueror sank an Argentine Navy light cruiser, General Belgrano, killing 323 Argentine Navy men, the Sun broke the news with the tasteless headline: "GOTCHA."

"Where exactly are the Falkland Islands?" I asked with genuine curiosity as we sat in the doctors' lounge after a hard day's work.

Were these islands located off the Welsh coast or were they in the English Channel between the UK and Europe? Nobody seemed to know. It was April 2, 1982, the day Argentina "invaded" the Falklands. The anchor on the evening news broadcast soon clarified our doubt. The Falkland Islands was an archipelago located in the South

Atlantic Ocean off the coast of Argentina nearly 8,000 miles from the UK and yes, they belonged to Great Britain. (see Fig 4)

The demise of colonialism in the middle of the twentieth century led to extraordinary and often quixotic predicaments for ex-colonial powers. What should their attitude be towards small pockets of land in far-flung regions that had somehow escaped the tide of indigenous nationalism and were still under their control? Should they relinquish authority to contiguous local governments or hold on to them?

Often, they chose to hold on to these lands against all sane advice and against all logistic geographical persuasion. Goa in India was a classic example of the stubbornness exhibited by ex-colonial powers – Portugal being the colonial power in that case.

Goa is a picturesque region located along the west coast of India, about 350 miles south of Mumbai, well known for its beaches. It spans an area of approximately 1,500 square miles and is one of modern India's smaller states. In the 1500s the Portuguese landed in Goa and took control of the region, holding onto it even as the rest of India came under British occupation.

In 1947, when the British finally vacated India, the logical thing for Portugal to do would have been to withdraw from Goa in deference to the strong nationalistic sentiment that was sweeping the region. But Portugal would have none of it. Portugal refused to give up Goa despite the peaceful exhortations of Indian leaders.

Eventually, after waiting nearly 14 years for a spontaneous change of heart on the part of the Portuguese, on December 19, 1961 India sent a small armed force into Goa that sent the Portuguese packing back to Lisbon. In an action that lasted about 48 hours and resulted in minimal casualties, India ended 451 years of Portuguese rule in Goa.

I am tempted to call the Falklands episode as Britain's Goa moment. But the comparison may not be entirely accurate. While the scenario was similar in terms of the distance between the mother country and the dependent territory, there was a difference in the identities of the combatants. The Falklands dispute was a confrontation between two colonial powers. Argentina was not a pristine, indigenous polity. Strictly speaking it was a country that traced its origin to the Spanish occupation of South America and was a creation of Spanish conquistadores. Its suzerainty over the islands was based on the claim that it had inherited the Malvinas (as they called them) from the Spanish monarchy. Argentina's strongest claim to the Falkland Islands rested on its geographical proximity: the islands are located 250 nautical miles off the coast of Argentina, rather than on any accurate historical proof.

The British reaction to the invasion was more emotional than cerebral. It lacked a sane objective assessment of the situation based on long-term consequences or logistic issues. It may even have been political. Prime Minister Margaret Thatcher was passing through difficult times and needed something to galvanize the nation and shore up her waning popularity. The Falklands situation presented her with the ideal opportunity. In hindsight, some political commentators even wonder whether she would have been re-elected with such an overwhelming victory (a 144-seat majority) in 1983 had it not been for the Falklands War.

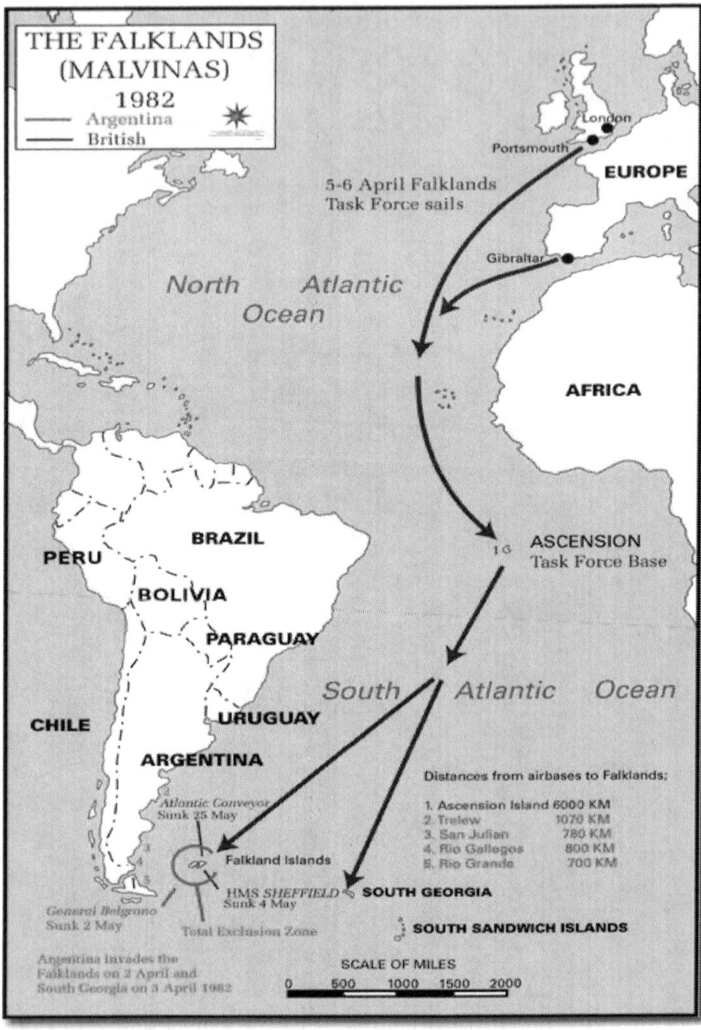

Fig.4. Map showing the Falkland Islands and their distance from Britain

There was however a definite element of imperialism driving the response. Margaret Thatcher turned this seemingly nondescript event – the takeover of a remote group of islands inhabited by no more than 3,000 people – into an issue of national importance and national destiny. The famous Argentinean writer Jorge Luis Borges aptly dubbed the Falklands War as "a fight between two bald men over a comb."

But Margaret Thatcher saw it differently. In her book, *The Downing Street Years,*she writes:

> "*Nothing remains more vividly in my mind, looking back on my years in 10 Downing Street, than the eleven weeks in the spring of 1982 when Britain fought and won the Falklands War. Much was at stake: what we were fighting for eight thousand miles away in the South Atlantic was not only the territory and the people of the Falklands, important though they were. We were defending our honor as a nation, and principles of fundamental importance to the whole world - above all that aggressors should never succeed and that international law should prevail over the use of force. The war was very sudden. No one predicted the Argentine invasion more than a few hours in advance, though many predicted it in retrospect. When I became Prime Minister I never thought that I would have to order British troops into combat and I do not think I have ever lived so tensely or intensely as during the whole of that time.*
>
> *The significance of the Falklands War was enormous, both for Britain's self-confidence and for our standing in the world. Since the Suez fiasco*

> *in 1956, British foreign policy had been one long retreat. The tacit assumption made by British and foreign governments alike was that our world role was doomed steadily to diminish. We had come to be seen by both friends and enemies as a nation which lacked the will and the capability to defend its interests in peace, let alone in war.*"

Thatcher's attitude, right from the beginning, was like that of a medieval ruler and every word she uttered in her feisty voice sounded like a battle cry. Pragmatism was missing. The result: the country found itself in the frenzied grip of jingoism. I saw a crude, vulgar display of antipathy everywhere in the country: among my physician colleagues who broke out into a loud applause every time an enemy vessel was targeted, in the talk among the common people on the street, and in the news media, both print and TV.

The Sun, a tabloid newspaper, assumed a singularly notorious role, arrogating to itself the voice of the country and becoming the official cheerleader for Margaret Thatcher. One headline read: "Stick it up your Junta." On another occasion, when the Royal Navy submarine HMS Conqueror sank an Argentine Navy light cruiser, General Belgrano, killing 323 Argentine Navy men, the Sun broke the news with the tasteless headline: "GOTCHA." (see Fig.5)

Though the public response to such headlines was mixed, they did appropriately capture the mood of the nation. The image of the civilized Englishman with a stiff upper lip that I had carried in my mind took a severe beating. There was an ugly side to him and the Falklands War exposed his deficiencies for all to see.

This unbridled jingoism seemed to prepare the ground for a military assault, leaving little room for peaceful negotiations. A task force was put together and set sail for the Falklands soon after April 2. The size of the task force – more than 100 ships – was excessive for the job at hand and conjured up an image of using a sledgehammer to swat a fly.

Two things about the war still stand out in my memory. One was the sinking of the Argentinean cruiser *General Belgrano*on on May 2, an event that was shrouded in much controversy and an action that Margaret Thatcher called "one of the most decisive military actions of the war." That it was a decisive action there is little doubt. With the sinking of the *Belgrano*, the Argentine Navy was completely paralyzed and posed no further danger to the British Armed Forces during the remainder of the operation. Additionally, on the diplomatic front, this attack proved beneficial. It thwarted a Peruvian peace initiative and allowed Britain to successfully achieve its military objective that it was dead set upon.

There was also some disagreement about the legality of the attack as it had occurred outside the 200-mile exclusion zone. However, the most disturbing aspect was the loss of human lives: 323 Argentinean sailors died in the attack. It signaled the first human casualties of the war and made peaceful negotiations almost impossible.

The other thing related to the war that I can recall is the *Exocet*missile. The *Exocet*is an anti-ship missile built by France and Argentina had supposedly acquired five of these. Powerful and precise, with radar-eluding capabilities, the *Exocet* had the potential to be a game-changer. The Royal Navy was very nervous and media hype had made the *Exocet* almost a household word in Britain during the war.

The first use of an *Exocet*missile by Argentina came on May 4, two days after the sinking of the *Belgrano*. The British destroyer HMS *Sheffield*was struck by an *Exocet* missile and incapacitated, and 20 British sailors were killed in the process. Back in Britain the mood turned somber but also vengeful. Cries for blood filled the air. From then on, there was no turning back.

Finally, on June 14, nearly 11 weeks after the Argentinean invasion, and after overcoming serious hostilities, British forces retook the islands and reestablished British authority. In terms of human lives, the cost was enormous: 904 in all, 649 Argentine and 255 British.

Speaking to Parliament after the victory, Margaret Thatcher emphasized what had been the driving forces beneath this violent exercise: imperialism and triumphalism:

> "*We have ceased to be a nation in retreat. We have instead a new-found confidence – born in the economic battles at home and tested and found true 8,000 miles away. That confidence comes from the re-discovery of ourselves, and grows with the recovery of our self-respect. And so today, we can rejoice at our success in the Falklands and take pride in the achievement of the men and women of our Task Force. But we do so, not as at some last flickering of a flame which must soon be dead. No – we rejoice that Britain has re-kindled that spirit which has fired her for generations past and which today has begun to burn as brightly as before. Britain found herself again in the South Atlantic*

and will not look back from the victory she has won."

Although this was seemingly a confident victory speech, Mrs Thatcher's choice of the phrase, "the last flickering of a flame" subconsciously and paradoxically expressed what the Falklands War really was: the last pathetic assertion of a waning colonial power.

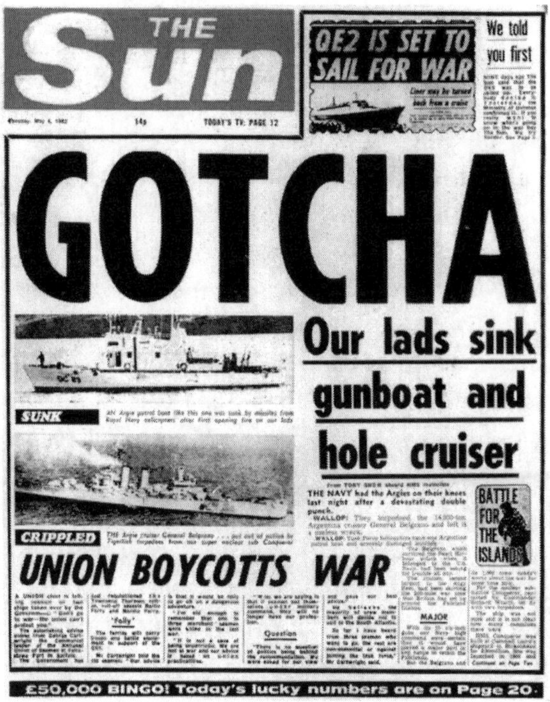

THE Sun

14p

TODAY'S TV: PAGE 12

QE2 IS SET TO SAIL FOR WAR

We told you first

GOTCHA

Our lads sink gunboat and hole cruiser

SUNK

CRIPPLED

THE NAVY had the Argies on their knees last night after a devastating double punch.

BATTLE FOR THE ISLANDS

UNION BOYCOTTS WAR

£50,000 BINGO! Today's lucky numbers are on Page 20.

Fig.5. Headlines in the The Sun

CHAPTER TWENTY-TWO

MRCP PART TWO AND DUBLIN

Thus, ended the saga of my second attempt at MRCP Part Two. I returned to South Shields dejected. Over the next few months, I found myself slipping into a black hole from which I saw no escape, a world of gloom and doom. More than two years after I landed in the UK, I seemed to be exactly where I had started. In practical terms I had made no headway in finding a way into the US. True, I had passed all the required exams, but with no appropriate visa and no offer of a residency position, everything that I had done so far amounted to naught. My repeated failures in the MRCP exams only added to my consternation. My worst fear appeared to be rapidly turning into a reality. I became convinced that I would never get to the US.

My first visit to Dublin to appear for Part One of the MRCP exam had been a hurried one. I landed in Dublin the night before the exam and went to bed almost immediately.

The next morning, I woke up, grabbed a quick breakfast and rushed to the examination hall. And around 12 noon after answering the 60 multiple-choice questions that were asked of me, I headed straight back to the airport. In less than 24 hours, I was back in South Shields. I had no time to take in the sights of Dublin or indulge in a meaningful interaction with the local population.

My later visits to Dublin provided me with a little more time to look around Dublin. The Part Two exam, as I mentioned earlier, was a day-long affair consisting of a written-cum-oral component in the morning followed by a clinical test in the afternoon that was contingent on one passing the first section. The clinical exam was a daunting affair. It brought one face to face with real patients and involved a direct confrontation with a human examiner. It was not only a test of one's medical knowledge: it called into play one's cognitive skills, the ability to remain calm under stress, and the ability to think clearly and quickly within a limited time frame. So, it was normal for the examinees to arrive a day or two earlier. It gave one time to unwind, settle in and prepare mentally for the ordeal.

In my first attempt at Part Two, I was a miserable failure. I didn't get past the first round. The written test was not difficult and I did fairly well. But the *viva voce* or oral component proved to be my stumbling block. In hindsight, the clinical quiz that had me groping for an answer was relatively simple, meriting nothing more than a little common sense. Yet overcome by a bout of panic, I failed to respond with the right answer.

The examiner, an aging Irishman with silver-gray hair and a thick Irish accent had this condescending air about him that had made me a little edgy to start with. His first question was quite easy and concerned a chest X-ray that depicted an obvious pneumothorax (air in the pleural cavity). It was an exact replica of Derek's chest X-ray. Derek, if you recollect, was my patient in South Shields in whom I had hesitatingly inserted a chest tube, my first, to relieve the pneumothorax that was hampering his breathing.

This is a case of pneumothorax, I responded confidently pointing out the clear lucency bereft of lung tissue at the upper part of the lung that was suggestive of an air pocket overlying a collapsed lung. The follow-up question was the one that cooked my goose.

If the upper part of the lung was diseased by scarring and tacked down, where would you see the air, was the examiner's next query. It was obvious that the air would be displaced to the side or lower part of the lung. But something happened to me. I broke out into a sweat, my lips just wouldn't respond to my commands and I stared blankly at the examiner. The examiner waited for a whole minute and when he found no response forthcoming he dismissed me with the words, "Thank you, doctor. You may go."

I knew that I had failed. The confirmation came an hour later when the list of candidates who would proceed to the next phase of the exam was put up. My name was nowhere.

I returned to Dublin three months later in the summer of 1982. A few more months of preparation had given me an added sense of confidence. I was also calmer. I knew from my past experience what the exam entailed and was not unduly perturbed by it. Moreover, I made it a point to arrive in Dublin two days prior to my exam date in order to relax and temper my nerves.

The bed and breakfast that I checked into late one evening was a nondescript little place situated on a dark side-street a few blocks away from O'Connell Street, the main thoroughfare of Dublin. It appeared to be a council home that had been converted into a lodging establishment. I had been told by my colleagues who had stayed here earlier that this place catered mostly to the exam-going crowd of foreign physicians and was safe. A bright pink neon sign proclaimed to the world its name, *Hotel Belvedere*, a high-sounding name for a modest lodging. Anyway, it didn't matter to me. It was inexpensive and conveniently located.

The inside of the bed and breakfast appeared to be straight out of a Dickensian novel. It was dark and dingy. A musty odor hung in the air. I was met at the door by a bent-over, aging housekeeper who kept shuffling about and mumbling incoherently as she pointed me in the direction of a staircase that led up to a corridor on the first floor.

Along this windowless corridor were six rooms that made up the entire complement of "Hotel Belvedere." My room itself was no bigger than a closet with a sagging steel bed, a not-too-clean blanket and a cramped shower area. The dining room that I visited later that night had the same aura of decrepitude. Cobwebs dangled precariously from old chandeliers. Dust was everywhere: on the tables, the chairs and the curtains. The furniture creaked with every touch. A somber-looking reticent waiter served me a cold meal of soggy fried potatoes and boiled vegetables that could hardly be described as appetizing. I did manage, however, to get a good night's sleep as I was too tired to be affected by these surroundings.

Ever since my school days I have adhered to a strict personal code of conduct with regards to examinations: I refrain from opening my books on the day prior to the exam, a ritual that I believe helps me perform better on the exam.

So, the next morning, my designated study-free day, after a quick breakfast of fried eggs, cold cereal and a glass of orange juice I ventured into the streets of Dublin – or onto O'Connell Street to be more specific.

I spent the greater part of that day on O'Connell Street, wandering aimlessly, observing people go by, peering through crystal-clear shop windows and pausing to take in the imposing architecture of the elegant stone buildings that lined the street or admire the statues that dotted the landscape. I even found an Indian restaurant tucked away on one of the side streets and indulged myself with a sumptuous meal of nan, *aloo gobi*, rice and dal. By the end of the day I had walked the entire length of O'Connell Street. It had been a satisfying outing.

My description of that day would be incomplete without mentioning an amusing incident that occurred. Sometime around late afternoon as I paused at a pedestrian crossing, I turned around to encounter a breathless young man bearing down on me. At first sight he appeared to be a fellow Indian but on closer scrutiny I detected some physical traits that suggested that I could be mistaken. He indicated that he had spotted me from across the street and had hurried to meet me. I am a Malaysian, he professed, clarifying my doubt, and then, in a tone that had desperation written all over it, proceeded to ask me, "Where can I find rice to eat?"

This was his first trip out of Malaysia, he explained. He had been staying in Dublin for a week and had been literally starving for he found the local food unpalatable. Tasteless, was his comment. Seeing me, an Indian, he was confident I would be able to help him. I gave him directions to the Indian restaurant that I had visited that afternoon.

Thanking me profusely and without wasting another minute, he dashed off in the direction of the restaurant to partake of a rice meal.

My second attempt at MRCP Part Two started off on a good note. The written part was relatively easy and did not throw up any unexpected questions. The oral component too did not prove to be too much of a hurdle and I easily sailed through to the clinical part.

The clinical test is conducted in a hospital and one's designated center could be any one of the numerous hospitals that were spread-out all-over Dublin. Luckily my locale proved to be close by and I reached there much ahead of the 2 PM start time.

The clinical component consisted of a series of short cases and one long case. The "short case" session was a walk-through experience with the examiner leading you from one patient to another in sequence. Each encounter involved a limited exam confined to one system like the heart or lungs followed by a summative diagnostic query. This exercise called for prompt clinical correlation. You had to get it right the first time around, within a minute or two. There was no second chance.

My first case was a young woman in her 30s with large bulging eyes and a prominent swelling in the neck. Thyrotoxicosis (increased activity of the thyroid gland), I declared confidently. Next, the examiner beckoned me to listen to the heart of a young boy: mitral stenosis (narrowing of the heart valve) I replied without any hesitation. The third was an elderly patient with deformed fingers: rheumatoid arthritis was my prompt response. I was on a roll. I answered correctly to two more questions. In all, I had five correct answers – the unofficial number for a pass in this section. The examiner deemed it unnecessary to quiz me on the remaining three patients. He waived me on to my long case.

The long case is a more detailed test of one's clinical skills. You are given one full hour to assess a patient, including taking a comprehensive history and performing a complete physical evaluation of all human body systems. I was given the case of a patient who had suffered a stroke.

After a brief review of my history-taking skills, the examiner asked me to perform a complete neurological examination in his presence. Midway he stopped me and asked me to demonstrate a 'knee-jerk' with the patient in the lying position. A knee-jerk is a simple exam that tests the integrity of the muscles and nerves of the leg. A tap on the tendon below the knee in normal individuals produces an extension of the leg, hence the term knee-jerk. There is a method to performing this test: the angle to which the leg has to be raised and the manner in which it needs to be supported prior to tapping the tendon are crucial to getting the correct response. A lapse in any of these prerequisites is sufficient to make one fail the exam. So, when the examiner asked me to repeat the test one more time after my first effort, I knew I was in trouble. There appeared to be a deficiency, real or imagined, in my technique according to the examiner. Again, he barked after my second attempt and I knew I had failed. Without even waiting for me to complete my examination, he walked away leaving me crestfallen.

Thus, ended the saga of my second attempt at MRCP Part Two. I returned to South Shields dejected. Over the next few months, I found myself slipping into a black hole from which I saw no escape, a world of gloom and doom. More than two years after I landed in the UK, I seemed to be exactly where I had started. In practical terms I had made no headway in finding a way into the US. True, I had passed all the required exams, but with no appropriate visa and no offer of a residency position, everything that I had done so far amounted to naught. My repeated failures in the MRCP exams only added to my consternation. My worst fear appeared to be rapidly turning into a reality. I became convinced that I would never get to the US.

About two months after my second attempt, and when I thought that things couldn't get worse, they did. I found myself facing the prospect of unemployment once again. My term as an SHO in the chest unit at South Shields was coming to an end. Despite Herculean efforts I had not been able to secure another job. My pleas to my consultant to give me another extension had been met with the cold retort that more than three extensions were not given. I couldn't help but interpret this reaction as payback for my intemperate behavior. Anyway, there was precious little that I could do about this.

Being unemployed as a junior physician in the UK brought with it more mundane travails. It meant being homeless as well: housing came with the job. No job meant no place to stay: I had to vacate my apartment. Where would I go? Where would I stay? These were the thoughts that haunted me in the last few days of my tenure in the chest unit.

As a last-ditch measure I approached the hospital administrator. I felt he owed me a good turn. I had helped him find locum candidates at short notice on several occasions. I was sure that he would be more sympathetic to my plight. But he too turned a deaf ear to my request.

Luckily a colleague of mine, Dr Sharma, who worked on the geriatric unit agreed to accommodate me in his room. Dr Sharma was at least 8 to 10 years older than me.

He had come to the UK after working in a few dead-end unsatisfying jobs in the eastern city of Kolkata (or Calcutta as it was then called). He was less ambitious than me and was happy to settle into a career in geriatrics.

His room was small, 10 feet long and 8 feet wide. It was meant for one person and could accommodate no more furniture than what was already there: a twin bed, a table and a chair. Built into the wall was a single closet that was already overflowing with Dr Sharma's belongings, leaving me no space to put mine. So, I piled my possessions into one corner of the room, pushed my suitcase underneath the bed and made myself as comfortable as I possibly could. I slept on a makeshift mattress of a few blankets that I spread out on the floor every night. It was a spartan arrangement, but I was happy to have a place to stay.

Despite these trying circumstances I soldiered on working towards my Part Two exam. In the summer of 1982 I returned to Dublin for what would be my third attempt. After two unsuccessful attempts I was neither excited nor nervous. I seemed to be fatalistically resigned to whatever outcome was slated for me.

I went through the ritual of the morning session without any hiccups. The afternoon clinical ordeal too appeared to pass off without any major drawbacks. I breezed through the short cases with ease. My short cases included a cirrhotic with a large belly, a patient with fluid around his lung (or a pleural effusion as it is medically termed), an elderly man with syphilis and a leaking heart valve (aortic insufficiency), a young woman with celiac diseases and typical skin blisters (dermatitis herpetiformis) on her shin and a middle-aged woman with facial paralysis or Bell's palsy.

My long-case examiner was a contrast to the surly worthy that I had encountered on my previous venture. He was friendlier, given to breaking into a smile frequently, more vocal and definitely more sympathetic to the plight of edgy examinees. He listened patiently to my presentation, observed me closely as I went through my examination and posed questions that would be classified as reasonable by any examinee. I walked out of the exam ward with some degree of satisfaction. But a pass was still not a guarantee. I had heard of too many instances in which candidates had mistaken an examiner's affability to mean approval, only to be disappointed when the results were announced. I would have to wait six more weeks to know my fate.

I got the news of my success when I was back in Walsall for an interview for a permanent registrar position. A colleague of mine from South Shields had taken the liberty to open my letter from the Royal College and called me up to give me the good news. I didn't get the registrar job in Walsall but passing the MRCP Part Two more than made up for my disappointment that day. But would it help me accomplish my ultimate goal?

CHAPTER TWENTY-THREE

A Locum Again: Back to Square One

I began to protest. How could I meet him at such short notice? I didn't have a travel visa to the US or an airline ticket to New York. To get these requirements completed in two working days, Thursday and Friday, seemed impossible. But Dr Bhowmick would have none of it. He gave me an ultimatum: "If you want this job, be here on Monday."

After one and a half years of relative stability, I plunged back into the world of uncertainty and locums. The classified advertisement section of the *BMJ* again became my focus; mailing out hundreds of résumés and expectant anxiety again became my routine. It was déjà vu all over again.

My prospects of getting to the US appeared to be bleaker than ever. The interview season for residencies beginning in July of 1983 was already in full swing in the US. With no interviews lined up, another fruitless year appeared to be in the offing. My next crack at a residency position would be two years down the road, July of 1984, eons away in my time frame. My ultimate goal appeared to be slowly but surely fading from the horizon.

More pressing at this time however was my daily sustenance, my food and lodging. I managed to land a seven-day locum as an SHO in the geriatrics department of South Shields General Hospital. Despite my strong aversion to working in geriatrics I had no choice but to accept the position as it would provide me with lodging for at least a week. After the geriatrics locum came a house officer position in medicine in a town called Barrow-in-Furness in Cumbria located in the northwest of the UK. I was slipping lower and lower in the hierarchy. But at this stage I really didn't care. I was too numbed to even react or comprehend the implications of this downturn. It meant another 10 days of paid accommodation and that was good enough for me. The only saving grace of this position was the train ride to Barrow-in-Furness. The train traversed through an area that was astoundingly beautiful: picturesque lakes dotted a pristine countryside. For a short time I was able to forget my misery.

In times of adversity, one's expectations drift lower. I found myself being thankful for small mercies. Landing a locum position to keep myself afloat became my pressing mission; my hunt for a permanent job temporarily receded to the background.

I have always believed that there is a very fine line between success and failure and one can never be certain when that line can be breached or how far or close to that line one is. Therefore, persistence is key, regardless of the apparent trajectory of one's fortunes. Change can occur in a few days or even a few moments and in a flash one's seemingly overwhelming travails are relegated to a footnote in one's life.

When I had all but given up hope of making it to the US, things changed. In a span of 10 days in early January 1983 my fortunes took an upward turn. After attending umpteen unsuccessful interviews for a registrar position, I finally landed one in Scarborough, a name that I was familiar with because of the 1960s hit song *Scarborough Fair*sung by Simon and Garfunkel. The song had become even more famous after featuring on the soundtrack of the blockbuster Dustin Hoffman movie, *The Graduate*.

Two days after getting the job in Scarborough which was slated to begin two months later in February, a friend of mine provided me with a lead that would prove invaluable. He had just returned from the US and advised me to call North General Hospital located in Harlem: the hospital was in need of residents for the term beginning in July 1983 and was willing to sponsor suitable candidates for a Green Card.

The sequence of events that followed is still clear in my mind, nearly three decades later. It was January 5, 1983, a Wednesday, when I called Dr Bhowmick, the program director at North General Hospital. By the brusque tone of his voice and his abrupt manner of speech I gathered that Dr Bhowmick was a no-nonsense man. He interrogated me for a full 15 minutes querying me about my experience and my credentials: the fact that I had passed the MRCP exam appeared to carry a lot of weight with him. At the end of the conversation he asked me to meet him in his office on Monday, January 10.

I began to protest. How could I meet him at such short notice? I didn't have a travel visa to the US or an airline ticket to New York. To get these requirements completed in two working days, Thursday and Friday, seemed impossible. But Dr Bhowmick would have none of it. He gave me an ultimatum: "If you want this job, be here on Monday." Without any further discussion, he hung up the phone.

Left with no choice, I traveled to Edinburgh to the US consulate the following day. My job offer from Scarborough General Hospital proved to be crucial, firming my belief in the notion that when you truly desire something, the entire universe will conspire to make it happen. The consular authorities were convinced that with a firm job offer I was less likely to remain behind in the US and granted me a travel visa without any hassle. On the morning of January 9, a Sunday, I flew out of Heathrow on my way to New York.

CHAPTER TWENTY-FOUR

CONCLUSION

Maybe my inner self had a sense of clairvoyance that my external faculties did not possess. Maybe my inner self knew that I had reached my destination and there was no going back to the UK.

I stood on the curb in front of the international arrivals building at JFK waiting to flag down another cab. A few minutes earlier, a taxi driver had picked me up, only to drop me off at the far end of the terminal where there was no police officer to berate him: his excuse was that the Bronx is a dangerous place to go at this time of the day. The shadows of evening were lengthening and darkness was setting in, making my chances of persuading another cab driver to embark on a journey to a seemingly scary Bronx even more difficult.

It was early January and biting cold. Small half-melted mounds of snow graced the edges of the curb, remnants of the snowstorm that had hit New York the week before. As usual I was clad in a coat that was too thin to protect me from the frigid temperature. Heavy icy air made breathing difficult. My teeth chattered incessantly. My naked fingers without the protective cover of gloves were becoming stiff. I rubbed my hands together feverishly to generate some heat and thrust them into my pockets for temporary respite. Puffs of air exuding my mouth formed visible clouds on the outside.

My friend who lived in the Bronx had agreed to put me up but had declined to come to the airport citing a work commitment. So, there was no one at the airport to receive me. The predicament that I faced now was no different from what I had experienced when I landed in London two years earlier.

Everything appeared unfamiliar and the future was still uncertain. The same questions plagued me. Would the interview go off well? Would I get the residency that I had applied for? And even if I did get the residency position, how would I get a Green Card, the ultimate proof of having arrived in the US? Would I have to go back to the UK?

Despite the myriad questions swirling around in my head I felt no anxiety this time. Strangely enough I felt an unusual calm on the inside which I found difficult to comprehend or explain. Maybe my inner self had a sense of clairvoyance that my external faculties did not possess. Maybe my inner self knew that I had reached my destination and there was no going back to the UK.

A yellow cab lumbered to a halt in front of me. I opened the door and slid into the back seat.

"Where to?" the driver asked without turning around.

"233rd street in the Bronx," I replied. The cab accelerated, picked up speed and eased into the traffic making its way into the greatest city in the world.

Glossary

Asian: In the UK, Asian refers to Indians, Pakistanis and Bangladeshis.

Residency:after completion of medical school, graduates in the US are required to undergo a supervised training program which may vary from three to five years depending on the specialty prior to being licensed to practice independently.

Internship: first year of the residency program.

Intern: physician doing internship.

Attending: a fully trained physician who has completed a residency or fellowship.

Consultant: fully trained physician in the UK, equivalent of an attending in the US.

House Officer: training grade in the UK equivalent to an intern.

Senior House Officer (SHO): training grade in the UK, higher than a house officer.

Registrar:training grade above an SHO.

Senior Registrar: above a registrar, stepping stone to a consultant.

MRCP: Member of the Royal College of Physicians.

FRCS: Fellow of the Royal College of Surgeons.

Geriatrics: specialty of medicine that deals with diseases of the elderly.

General Medicine: General or internal medicine is a medical specialty that deals with the prevention, diagnosis and treatment of diseases in adults. Usually does not involve surgical operations.

NHS: National Health Service, the agency responsible for healthcare in the UK.

PLAB: Professional and Linguistic Assessments Board.

USMLE: The United States Medical Licensing Examination.

Underground: Subway.

Tube Station: Subway station.